£11.95

CASE STUDIES IN

ST BARTHOLOMEW'S AND THE ROYAL LON
SCHOOL OF MEDICINE AND DENTISTRY
LIBRARY, ... STREET, LONDO

PATHOLOGY

Alan Stevens MBBS, FRCPath

and

Jim Lowe BMedSci, BMBS, DM, MRCPath

Department of Histopathology
Queen's Medical Centre
University Hospital NHS Trust
Nottingham, UK

M Mosby

London Baltimore Bogotá Boston Buenos Aires Caracas Carlsbad, CA Chicago Madrid Mexico City Milan Naples, FL
New York Philadelphia St. Louis Sydney Tokyo Toronto Wiesbaden

Project Manager:	Jonathan Brenchley
	Louise Cook
Developmental Editor:	Rachael Miller
Designer/Layout Artist:	Louise Bond
Cover Design:	Pete Wilder
Production:	Jane Tozer
Index:	Nina Boyd
Publisher:	Fiona Foley

PREFACE

We believe that a breadth of knowledge of pathology is essential for good clinical diagnostic and management skills in hospital, office, family and/or community practice. This case studies book is designed to complement our student text book *Pathology* to which each case is cross referenced. Cases are presented which highlight important areas of pathology and relate these to clinical diagnosis and patient management. We hope that you enjoy the cases and that they make some aspects of pathology memorable.

The names used throughout the book, together with the clinical histories, are entirely contrived and any resemblance to any person living or dead is purely coincidental.

We would like to thank our contributors for their unstinting efforts in assisting in the compilation of this book. Any errors are our own and not theirs.

AS
JL
Nottingham 1994

CONTRIBUTORS

Richard Allibone MB ChB, BSc, MRCPath
Margaret Balsitis MB ChB, MRCPath
Zia Choudry MB ChB, MSc
Helen Goulding BA, MB BS, MRCPath
Gill Kirk BSc, MB ChB
Iain Leach MB ChB, DM
Paul Matthews MB BS, BSc
Sarah Pinder MB ChB, MRCPath
Rachel Sheeran BSc, MB ChB, PhD

From the Departments of Histopathology, University
and City Hospitals, Nottingham, UK.

Clinical Editor
Matthew Jackson MB BS, MRCP
Department of Neurology, Queen's Medical Centre,
University Hospital NHS Trust, Nottingham, UK.

CONTENTS

BLOOD CIRCULATORY SYSTEM

CASE 1

Frederick Polson, a 65-year-old retired truck driver, is admitted to hospital because of the sudden onset of severe pain affecting most of his right leg. He had recently retired as a truck driver. On examination, the leg is cold and pale; he is in sinus rhythm and the femoral pulse is present though weak, but the distal pulses are absent. He has been a life-long cigarette smoker and has a three-year history of angina and atrial fibrillation, and a five-year history of intermittent claudication in the right leg.

Questions

1 What disease process underlies this patient's chronic symptoms?
2 What are the main risk factors predisposing to this disease process?
3 What are the two possible explanations for his acute symptoms?

YOUR ANSWERS

1 Disease process underlying this patient's chronic symptoms

ATHEROMA → ATHEROSCLEROSIS.

2 Main risk factors predisposing to this disease process

CONSTITUTIONAL - Age, sex, Familial.
HARD · ↑ lipid, ↑Bp, DM, Smoking
SOFT - Exercise, overweight, stress

3 Two possible explanations for his acute symptoms

Thromboembolism
Thrombotic occlusion.

CASE 2

William Bannister is a 60-year-old warehouse supervisor. He visits his local family practitioner because he has become worried about vague abdominal pain and backache that he has been experiencing for about six months. His friend, Joe, has just been told he has cancer, and this was what made William go to see a doctor. He smokes 20 cigarettes a day, and has done so since he started work at the age of 14, but is otherwise well. On examination, his doctor notes a large pulsatile abdominal mass. An abdominal aortic aneurysm is diagnosed and he is referred to hospital for consideration of surgical intervention.

Questions

1 What is the likely cause of this patient's aneurysm?
2 Describe the histological changes occuring in the wall of the aorta in this condition?
3 What complications may occur?
4 What are the other main types of aneurysm and their causes?

YOUR ANSWERS

1 Likely cause of this patient's aneurysm

ATHEROSCLEROTIC

2 Histological changes occuring in the wall of the aorta

Thinning + fibrous replacement of media.

3 Complications that may occur

Rupture . Thromboembolise → distal site.

4 Other main types of aneurysm and their causes

Syphilitic
Berry
Infective.

CASE 1 ANSWERS

pp. 131, 132, 134, 144

1 Disease process underlying this patient's chronic symptoms

The disease process underlying this patients previous symptoms of angina and intermittent claudication is atheroma. Narrowing of one or more coronary arteries by atheroma results in insufficient myocardial blood flow during exercise and the symptoms of angina. Similarly, narrowing of the arteries to the lower limbs produces ischaemia of the muscles of the leg during exercise, leading to the symptoms of intermittent claudication.

2 Main risk factors predisposing to this disease process

The main risk factors for development of atheroma are:
- Hypercholesterolaemia.
- Hypertension.
- Diabetes mellitus.
- Cigarette smoking.
- Other possible contributory factors include lack of exercise, obesity, 'stress' and certain personality traits.

3 Two possible explanations for his acute symptoms

His acute symptoms are due to the sudden onset of severe ischaemia of the leg due to complete arterial occlusion. The two main possible causes for this are:
- Thromboembolism arising from the left atrium, with atrial fibrillation as a predisposing factor to thrombus formation in the atrial appendage, and reversion to sinus rhythm precipitating separation of the thrombus to form a thromboembolus.
- Thrombotic occlusion of the femoral artery, secondary to underlying atheroma.

CASE 2 ANSWERS

pp. 130, 133

1 Likely cause of this patient's aneurysm

Abdominal aortic aneurysms are caused by atheroma. Severe atheroma weakens the aortic media, allowing dilatation and the formation of aneurysm. Atheroma is generally most severe in the distal abdominal aorta and most aneurysms develop distal to the origin of the renal arteries.

2 Histological changes occuring in the wall of the aorta

The histological changes of atheroma are:
- Deposition of lipid in the intima of the vessel wall, some in myointimal cells and some free.
- Production of collagenous fibrosis in the intima.
- Loss of elastic and replacement of the muscle of the vessel wall by collagen.
- Thrombus formation in the aneurysm cavity.

3 Complications that may occur

Occasionally, atheroma debris or thrombus from within the aneurysm sac may embolise, producing distal arterial occlusion. The most serious complication is rupture of the aneurysm, leading to massive retroperitoneal haemorrhage, which usually proves rapidly fatal. Because of this, repair of larger (>5 cm) aneurysms using a Dacron graft is indicated.

4 Other main types of aneurysm and their causes
- Syphilitic aneurysms of the ascending aorta and arch are due to inflammatory destruction of the media, but nowadays are rare.
- Berry aneurysms affect the intracerebral arteries and are caused by a congenital defect in the vessel wall.
- Mycotic aneurysms are caused by inflammatory destruction of the vessel wall by bacteria within infected thromboemboli.
- Occasionally, aneurysms may develop secondary to a vasculitis as in polyarteritis nodosa or Kawasaki's disease.
- Note: dissecting aortic aneurysm is not a true aneurysm, but is a longitudinal dissection through the aortic media secondary to degeneration of the media.

CASE 3

Mrs Catherine Portman, a 36-year-old, recently divorced traffic warden, has been diagnosed as having gallstones after complaining of intermittent upper abdominal pain for just over a year. She is admitted to hospital for an elective cholecystectomy. She is obese, but is otherwise well, and is on no medication apart from the oral contraceptive pill. Three days after the operation she complains of right-sided chest pain, made worse by coughing, and slight shortness of breath. On examination, she has a right-sided pleural rub; her left calf is swollen, tender and warm, with pitting ankle oedema. Chest X-ray shows an ill-defined shadow in the right lower zone of the lung.

Questions

1 What is the diagnosis?
2 What factors predispose to this condition?
3 What are the other possible consequences of this condition?

YOUR ANSWERS

1 Diagnosis

PE following DVT.

2 Factors predisposing to this condition

Recent Surgery, Immobility, OCP, Pregnancy, Trauma, Burns, Cardiac failure, Nephrotic syndrome.

3 Other possible consequences of condition

Pulmonary embolus.

CASE 4

Harold de Bonville is a 58-year-old art historian. He was once an academic, but is now employed as a valuation expert at a large fine-art auction house. He has a seven-year history of hypertension, treated by his family practitioner. His blood pressure is currently around 180/110 mmHg. He has been referred to the hospital clinic because his blood pressure is proving difficult to control. Clinical examination is unremarkable; blood pressure is 185/115 mmHg. Results of investigations are shown below. His white cell count is normal.

Investigation	Result
Chest X-ray	Mild cardiac enlargement, lung fields clear
ECG	Left axis deviation, deep S waves V1–2, tall R waves V5–6, inverted T waves V5–6
Haemoglobin	12.0 g/dl, normocytic, normochromic
White-cell count	Normal
Urea	Mild elevation
Creatinine	Mild elevation
Sodium	Normal
Potassium	Normal
Phosphate	Normal
Serum albumin	Normal

Questions

1 What are the main causes of hypertension?
2 What are the main complications of hypertension?
3 What complications are suggested in this patient by the results of the investigations?

YOUR ANSWERS

1 Main causes of hypertension

1° - Idiopathic.
2°

2 Main complications of hypertension

LVF *AAA.*
Intracerebral haemorrhage
Benign hypertensive nephrosclerosis.

3 Complications suggested by the results of the investigations

LVF or hypertrophy.
Renal failure.

CASE 3 ANSWERS pp. 126, 127

1 Diagnosis
Deep leg-vein thrombosis with pulmonary thromboembolism and pulmonary infarction.

2 Factors predisposing to this condition
- Immobility and bed rest.
- Post-operative period.
- Pregnancy and the post-partum period.
- Oral contraceptives, though less so nowadays with current low dose oestrogen preparations.
- Nephrotic syndrome.
- Severe burns.
- Trauma.
- Cardiac failure.
- Disseminated malignancy.

3 Other possible consequences of condition
The five main consequences of leg vein thrombosis and pulmonary thromboembolism are:
- Massive pulmonary embolism leading to rapid death (5%).
- Major pulmonary embolism which is often symptomatic (10%).
- Minor pulmonary embolism which is frequently asymptomatic (85%).
- Recurrent minor pulmonary thromboemboli may lead to obliteration of the vascular bed and to pulmonary arterial hypertension.
- Post-phlebetic syndrome - a painful, cyanotic indurated pigmented leg with tense ankle oedema, due to irreversible damage to venous valves in the affected leg.

CASE 4 ANSWERS pp. 135, 136

1 Main causes of hypertension
In the majority (>90%) of cases there is no obvious cause, so-called 'essential' hypertension. In less than 10% of cases, hypertension is secondary to another disease process:
- Renal disease - renal artery stenosis, diffuse renal disease, e.g. long-standing glomerulonephritis or pyelonephritis.
- Endocrine disorders - phaeochromocytoma, Cushing's syndrome, Conn's syndrome, thyroid disease, acromegaly.
- Coarctation of the aorta.
- Drugs - steroids.
- Vasculitides - polyarteritis nodosa.
- Alcohol.

2 Main complications of hypertension
The main complications of longstanding hypertension are:
- Heart – left ventricular hypertrophy, cardiac failure, coronary artery atheroma, ischaemic heart disease.
- Aorta – atheroma, aneurysms and dissection.
- Brain – intracerebral haemorrhage, cerebral microinfarcts.
- Kidney – arteriolosclerosis leading to diffuse ischaemic damage to glomeruli and eventual chronic renal failure.

3 Complications suggested by the results of the investigations
The ECG abnormalities suggest left-ventricular hypertrophy whilst the mild anaemia and raised urea and creatinine are indicative of impaired renal function.

CASE 5

Mr Sean Bolinski is a 50-year-old police officer in the vice squad. He presents with a nine-month history of intermittent chest pain. It first started when he had to chase a prostitute along an alley and has since occurred when he exerts himself; it is relieved by rest. He describes it as a tightness 'like someone standing on my chest' which is sometimes associated with an ache in the left arm. A clinical diagnosis of chronic stable angina is made. He is overweight and smokes 40 cigarettes daily. His blood pressure is 160/100 mmHg but otherwise clinical examination and routine investigations are normal.

Questions

1 What pathological changes are likely to be present to cause stable angina?
2 What other acute manifestations might this patient suffer in the future?
3 What advice and treatment would you consider for this patient?

YOUR ANSWERS

1 Pathological changes likely to be present to cause stable angina

2 Other acute manifestations this patient might suffer in the future

3 Advice and treatment you consider for this patient

CASE 6

Mrs Florence Cartermile is a 57-year-old woman who works part-time in a bar. She is admitted to hospital with a two-hour history of sudden-onset severe crushing central chest pain radiating to the neck and left arm. This started while she was cleaning the cellar just after a delivery of beer. She is nauseated and has vomited twice. On examination, she is pale and sweaty with a tachycardia but normal blood pressure. An ECG shows ST elevation in leads V4-6. Her chest X-ray is normal. The clinical diagnosis is acute myocardial infarction.

Questions

1 What pathological event leads to acute myocardial infarction?
2 What immediate treatment would you give?
3 What investigations would you perform to confirm the diagnosis?
4 What are the main acute complications of myocardial infarction?

YOUR ANSWERS

1 Pathological event leading to acute myocardial infarction

2 Immediate treatment

3 Investigations performed to confirm diagnosis

4 Main acute complications of myocardial infarction

CASE 5 ANSWERS p. 144

1 Pathological changes likely to be present to cause stable angina

Stable angina is caused by an imbalance between myocardial oxygen demand and oxygen supply. This is almost always caused by narrowing of one or more coronary arteries by a stable plaque of atheroma. In general, this needs to narrow the lumen by more than 50% of its diameter before clinical symptoms develop.

2 Other acute manifestations this patient might suffer in the future

This patient is now symptomatic and has clearly significant coronary-artery atheroma. Rupture of a plaque, with formation of overlying thrombus could occur in the future, leading to one of the acute manifestations of coronary artery disease, namely:

- Unstable angina.
- Acute myocardial infarction.
- Sudden death.

3 Advice and treatment you would consider in this patient

After explaining the cause of his symptoms he should be advised to lose weight and must stop smoking. The symptoms of angina may be relieved by avoiding exertion to the point where symptoms are known to occur. Sublingual glyceryl trinitrate may be used prophylactically or to alleviate symptoms; various other oral drugs are available for more severe symptoms. His hypertension is a risk factor for atheroma, and also increases left-ventricular workload and should therefore be treated if it does not improve with weight loss alone.

Referral for investigation of coronary arteries by imaging with a view to angioplasty or an arterial bypass procedure should be considered.

CASE 6 ANSWERS pp. 145, 146, 148

1 Pathological event leading to acute myocardial infarction

Acute myocardial infarction is usually related to ulceration or fissuring of an atheromatous plaque within one of the coronary arteries, leading to thrombus formation and coronary artery occlusion.

2 Immediate treatment

- Pain relief and antiemetics.
- Administration of a thrombolytic drug such as streptokinase or tissue plasminogen activator and aspirin can lyse the thrombus, re-establishing blood flow and limiting the size of the infarct. This may reduce the severity of complications and improve survival.
- Further therapy depends on whether or not further complications arise.

3 Investigations performed to confirm diagnosis

Acute myocardial infarction is diagnosed clinically by demonstrating a rise in cardiac enzymes and/or by demonstrating specific changes on the ECG.

4 Main short-term complications of myocardial infarction

- Arrhythmias.
- Left-ventricular failure and pulmonary oedema.
- Rupture of the infarcted ventricular myocardium.
- Mitral-valve papillary dysfunction or rupture.
- Mural thrombus and systemic thromboembolism.
- Acute pericarditis.
- Deep-vein thrombosis and pulmonary thromboembolism.

CASE 7

Mr Julian Forbes is a 45-year-old wine bar owner. He has previously been in good health, but now presents with increasing shortness of breath on exertion to the point where he now becomes breathless climbing a flight of stairs. On examination, he is in atrial fibrillation and has scattered crepitations in both lung fields. Heart sounds are normal, with no murmurs, and his blood pressure is also normal. JVP is raised, and there is bilateral ankle oedema. The liver is impalpable. The results of investigations are shown below.

Investigation	Result
Haemoglobin	Macrocytic anaemia
Urea and electrolytes	Normal
γ-glutamyl transferase	Raised
Alanine aminotransferase	Raised
Alkaline phosphatase	Normal
Bilirubin	Normal
Serum albumin	Normal
Uric acid	Raised
Random blood glucose	Normal
Thyroid-function tests	Normal
ECG	Atrial fibrillation
Chest X-ray	Markedly enlarged heart
Echocardiogram	All four chambers dilated with globally-poor myocardial contractility; mild tricuspid and mitral regurgitation; valves morphologically normal
Coronary angiography	Normal coronary arteries
Blood film	Round macrocytosis and target cells

Clinically, he is diagnosed as having a dilated cardiomyopathy.

Questions

1 What is the evidence to support this diagnosis?
2 What are the main causes of dilated cardiomyopathy?
3 What is the most likely cause in this patient?

YOUR ANSWERS

1 Evidence to support diagnosis

2 Main causes of dilated cardiomyopathy

3 Most likely cause in this patient

CASE 7 ANSWERS

pp. 149, 150

1 Evidence to support diagnosis

The patient's symptoms and physical signs are due to combined left- and right-ventricular failure. He has a dilated heart with poor myocardial function. Investigations have shown normal blood pressure, coronary arteries and valves that effectively rules out hypertensive heart disease, ischaemic heart disease and valvular heart disease (the mitral and tricuspid regurgitation noted on echocardiography is secondary to the dilated ventricles). The most likely diagnosis is therefore dilated cardiomyopathy.

2 Main causes of dilated cardiomyopathy

The main causes of secondary dilated cardiomyopathy are:
- Multisystem disorders such as diabetes, thyroid disease, haemochromatosis and amyloid.
- Inflammatory diseases such as viral myocarditis.
- Toxic and metabolic causes such as alcohol and certain drugs.
- Muscular dystrophies and mitochondrial cytopathies.

In primary dilated cardiomyopathy the cause is unknown although some may be related to a previous subclinical episode of viral myocarditis.

3 Most likely cause in this patient

This patient's occupation, together with a macrocytic anaemia with round cells and abnormal liver function tests and raised urate, should raise a strong suspicion that alcohol abuse is the underlying cause.

CASE 8

Mrs Sheila Gordon is 39-year-old woman who lives above her TV repair shop with her husband and family. She is referred to hospital with a five-year history of increasing shortness of breath on exertion. She has a persistent cough and has had several episodes of slight haemoptysis. As a child, she had an episode of rheumatic fever. On examination, she is in sinus rhythm and has a loud first heart sound and a soft, apical diastolic murmur. Her chest is clear. Investigations show the following:

Investigation	Result
ECG	Sinus rhythm, prominent bifid P waves best seen in lead II
Chest X-ray	Prominent pulmonary veins, no obvious pulmonary oedema
Echocardiogram	Mitral stenosis with a dilated left atrium

You make a clinical diagnosis of mitral-valve stenosis.

Questions

1 What is the pathogenesis of mitral-valve stenosis?
2 What pathological abnormalities would you expect to see affecting the valve?
3 What are the main effects and complications of mitral stenosis?

YOUR ANSWERS

1 Pathogenesis of mitral-valve stenosis

2 Pathological abnormalities expected to be see affecting valve

3 Main effects and complications of mitral stenosis

CASE 9

Mr Tim Bourke is the 60-year-old headmaster of a boys school. He presents with a six-month history of chest pains which are suggestive of angina. He has recently started to become quite short of breath on exertion and has had two episodes of syncope, both associated with exertion. On examination, the most notable finding is a loud, ejection-systolic murmur, loudest in the aortic area, radiating into the carotids and associated with a palpable thrill. He has previously been fit and well and is not on any medication.

Questions

1 What is the diagnosis?
2 What are the main causes of this condition?
3 What are the main effects of this lesion?

YOUR ANSWERS

1 Diagnosis

2 Main causes of condition

3 Main effects of lesion

CASE 8 ANSWERS
p. 152

1 Pathogenesis of mitral-valve stenosis

Mitral stenosis is almost always a consequence of acute rheumatic fever, although a definite clinical history is not always obtained. Rheumatic fever usually occurs during childhood, and follows a streptococcal pharyngitis. Antibodies raised against bacterial antigens then cross-react with cardiac antigens producing a pancarditis. Inflammation of the valves is the most important component, as valvular inflammation leads to fibrosis and scarring of the valve, which in turn leads to valve dysfunction. Although acute rheumatic fever is now uncommon in most Western countries, there are still many patients with chronic rheumatic heart disease.

2 Pathological abnormalities expected to be seen affecting the valve

Chronic rheumatic mitral valve disease is characterized by:
- Fibrosis and thickening of the valve leaflets.
- Fusion of the valve commissures.
- Fibrosis and fusion of the chordae tendinae.
- Calcification of the leaflets.

These changes combine to produce a characteristic slit-like narrowed valve orifice.

3 Main effects and complications of mitral stenosis

- An increase in left-atrial pressure with left-atrial hypertrophy and dilatation.
- An increase in pulmonary-venous pressure produces pulmonary congestion and oedema which in turn leads to symptoms of dyspnoea and haemoptysis.
- Increased pulmonary-venous pressure may eventually lead to right-ventricular hypertrophy and right-heart failure.
- Left-atrial dilatation may lead to atrial fibrillation and left-atrial thrombosis with systemic thromboembolism.
- Thrombus formation on the valve may also lead to thromboembolism.
- Increased risk of developing infective endocarditis.

CASE 9 ANSWERS
p. 153

1 Diagnosis

Aortic-valve stenosis.

2 Main causes of condition

The three commonest causes are:
- Calcification occurring in a congenital, bicuspid, aortic valve.
- Calcification occurring in a normal tricuspid, aortic valve ('senile' calcification).
- Chronic rheumatic aortic-valve disease.

Occasionally, valvar, subvalvar or supravalvar stenosis may occur as a congenital abnormality.

3 Main effects of lesion

Stenosis of the aortic valve develops slowly, and cardiac output is initially maintained by compensatory left-ventricular hypertrophy. Angina is related to a mismatch between coronary blood flow and the oxygen requirements of the hypertrophied myocardium (some patients may also have coexistent coronary-artery atheroma). Syncope is thought to be due to inappropriate peripheral vasodilatation on exertion, secondary to abnormal left-ventricular baroreceptor responses. Pateints with syncope will often die within two years if untreated. Dyspnoea in patients with aortic stenosis is an ominous symptom; it signifies left-ventricular decompensation and the onset of left-ventricular failure. Sudden death due to cardiac arrhythmias is not uncommon in aortic stenosis, and may be the presenting 'symptom'.

CASE 10

Ms Fiona Bamworth is a 52-year-old woman who devises crossword puzzles for one of the national newspapers. She gives a six-week history of tiredness, lethargy, weight loss and intermittent fever and sweating. On examination she looks unwell, but is apyrexial. She has a left subconjunctival haemorrhage. A few petechiae are present over her legs and she has several splinter haemorrhages under her fingernails. Her spleen is just palpable. She has a tachycardia and a pansystolic murmur typical of mitral regurgitation. There is no definite history of rheumatic fever. Urine dipstick test is positive for blood The results of further investigations are shown below.

Investigation	Result
Haemoglobin	Mild normocytic, normochromic anaemia
White-cell count	Raised with a neutrophilia
ESR	Elevated
C-reactive protein	Raised
Urinalysis	Microscopic haematuria
Chest X-ray	Normal
Echocardiogram	Abnormal mitral valve with regurgitation but no definite vegetations
Blood cultures	*Streptococcus viridans* isolated from one of six pairs of blood cultures; sensitive to penicillin

A diagnosis of bacterial endocarditis is made and treatment with intravenous antibiotics is commenced.

Questions

1 What factors predispose to infective endocarditis?
2 What is the pathogenesis of the cardiac infective lesion?
3 What are the main complications?

YOUR ANSWERS

1 Factors predisposing to infective endocarditis

2 Pathogenesis of the cardiac infective lesion

3 Main complications

CASE 10 ANSWERS p. 154

1 Factors predisposing to infective endocarditis
Predisposing factors for infective endocarditis include:
- Congenital heart disease, especially patent ductus arteriosus, ventricular septal defect, coarctation of the aorta, Fallot's tetralogy and congenital bicuspid aortic valve.
- Acquired valvular heart disease, such as rheumatic heart disease and floppy mitral-valve disease.
- Prosthetic heart valves, intraventricular pacing wires.
- Intravenous drug abuse.
- Structurally normal valves may be infected by virulent organisms, for example in patients with infected bed sores.

2 Pathogenesis of the cardiac infective lesion
Numerous bacteria, fungi and other organisms can cause endocarditis. In general, low-virulence organisms such as *Streptococcus viridans* infect abnormal valves. A transient bacteraemia allows the bacteria to colonize platelet aggregates that overlie damaged endothelium or collect on prosthetic heart valves.

Virulent organisms such as *Staphylococcus aureus* or *Streptococcus pneumonia* may colonize apparently normal valves during an episode of septicaemia or bacteraemia. The duration of symptoms and the time scale of the illness are related to the virulence of the organism.

3 Main complications
The main complications can be divided into local and distant complications:
- Local destruction of the valve, producing incompetence of the valve and cardiac failure. This may occur within a few days with highly virulent organisms.
- Thromboemboli, which may produce widespread infarcts in other organs. If bacteria are present in these emboli, septic infarcts or mycotic aneurysms may occur.
- Immune-complex deposition produces the cutaneous petechiae and splinter haemorrhages, and may also lead to glomerulonephritis with haematuria.

2

RESPIRATORY SYSTEM

CASE 11

Mr Herbert Scuttle is 70-year-old retired postman. He has been admitted to hospital for transurethral resection of prostate under general anaesthesia. He has no significant past medical history and is on no medication. However, he has smoked 10 cigarettes a day for 40 years (20 pack-years). He undergoes an uneventful operation but is slow to mobilize post-operatively and, on the third day of his admission, complains of cough productive of yellow-green sputum.

On examination, he is pyrexial (temperature: 38.5°C) and has bilateral, coarse, expiratory crepitations.

He was commenced on amoxycillin pending the microbiology results. However, his symptoms worsened with production of increasing quantities of foul smelling sputum, a swinging pyrexia and confusional state. Following further investigation, *Klebsiella pneumoniae* was cultured; his antibiotic treatment was altered and he made a slow recovery.

Investigation	Result
Chest X-ray	Patchy opacities
White-cell count	Elevated neutrophil count
Haemoglobin	Normal
Urea and electrolytes	Normal
Blood culture	*Klebsiella pneumoniae* cultured

Questions

1 What is the most likely diagnosis for his initial symptoms?
2 What predisposing factors for the development of a chest infection did this man have?
3 Describe the pathological changes in the lungs?
4 What are the possible causes for the progression of his disease? What further investigations you would consider?

13

CASE 11 ANSWERS
pp. 154, 162–164

1 Most likely diagnosis for initial symptoms
The most likely diagnosis is a hospital-acquired pneumonia, defined as 'pneumonia occurring two days or more after admission to hospital'.

2 Predisposing factors for the development of a chest infection
This man had a reduced ability to clear bronchial secretions due to smoking, general anaesthesia and immobility – all predisposing him to infection by inhaled organisms.

3 Pathological changes in the lungs
He is likely to have a bronchopneumonia in which primary infection is centred on the bronchi and spreads to involve adjacent alveoli. Macroscopically, the lungs contain firm, airless areas which are dark red or grey in colour. Pus may be present in peripheral bronchi.

Microscopically, there is acute inflammation of bronchi and an acute inflammatory exudate in the alveoli. These features are most commonly seen in the dependent parts of the lungs, where retained secretions are more likely to gather.

4 Causes for progression of disease and further investigations
Most hospital-acquired pneumonia is caused by Gram-negative organisms. The antibiotic chosen for initial therapy, while reasonable for first-line treatment of a community-acquired chest infection, would not be the first-line choice for a hospital-acquired infection. Common complications of bronchopneumonia include pleurisy, septicaemia and lung abscess. It may be necessary to obtain an uncontaminated specimen of sputum by bronchoscopy and bronchial lavage in order to establish the cause of infection and antimicrobial sensitivity in severe cases that are unresponsive to therapy.

CASE 12

Mr George Burlington is a 25-year-old postdoctoral student studying Russian. He has presented with cough, wheeze and increasing respiratory distress developing gradually over about 12 hours. In between breaths he is able to describe similar attacks in the past, which he thought were precipitated by exercise and upper respiratory-tract infection, but never as bad as at present. He also has a history of atopic eczema and a sister who also suffered from childhood eczema. He is not taking any medication. On examination, he is pyrexial, tachycardic and centrally cyanosed. He has an expiratory wheeze with prolonged expiration.

He is treated with β-agonists and corticosteroids and makes a good recovery, but continues to suffer recurrent, similar but milder episodes, often precipitated by an upper respiratory-tract infection.

Investigation	Result
PEFR	Markedly reduced
FEV1/FVC	Reduced
PaO_2	7.0 kPa
$PaCO_2$	6.8 kPa
Chest X-ray	Hyperinflated chest with clear lung fields. No pneumothorax
White-cell count	Elevated with eosinophilia

Questions

1 What is the likely diagnosis and what further information would you obtain from the history?
2 What investigations would you perform to confirm the diagnosis and assess severity?
3 What do the results of the investigations given below indicate?
4 What is the structural basis for the clinical features and by what mechanisms do these occur?

YOUR ANSWERS

1 Likely diagnosis and further information from the history

2 Investigations performed to confirm diagnosis and assess severity

3 Indications of investigations

4 Structural basis for clinical features and mechanisms of occurrence

CASE 12 ANSWERS
pp. 159, 168–170

1 Likely diagnosis and further information from history
The most likely diagnosis is acute asthma. This is a very severe attack as indicated by the tachycardia, cyanosis and hypercapnia. Other information which may have been obtained from the history include other triggering factors such as drugs and occupational or domestic exposure to allergens, the most common being house dust containing dust-mite faeces.

2 Investigations to confirm diagnosis and assess severity
Initial investigations would include assessment of the peak expiratory flow rate (PEFR) which is reduced in asthma, and may improve following administration of β-agonists. The ratio of forced expiratory volume in 1 second to forced vital capacity (FEV1/FVC) is also reduced. A chest X-ray should also be performed. A full blood count may show a peripheral eosinophilia and serum IgE may be elevated. Sputum examination may identify Curschmann spirals and Charcot–Leyden crystals.

Signs of severe asthma include: central cyanosis, accessory muscle use with intercostal recession and tracheal tug, tachycardia (>150/min), tachypnoea (>28/min), and a forced expiratory time of more than four seconds.

3 Indications of investigations
The results in this case confirm a severe obstructive respiratory defect with type II respiratory failure. This is unusual in asthma and indicates a severe attack (status asthmaticus).

4 Structural basis for clinical features and pathogenesis
Increased responsiveness of the bronchial smooth muscle causes bronchoconstriction; mucosal oedema causes further narrowing. Obstruction to airflow is further exacerbated by hypersecretion of mucus causing mucus plugging. The mucus plugs may be seen in the sputum as Curschmann spirals. Infiltration of bronchial mucosa by inflammatory cells, including eosinophils, accounts for the presence of Charcot–Leyden crystals (which are derived from eosinophil granules) in the sputum. Other structural changes include focal necrosis of airway epithelium and subepithelial collagen deposition in long-standing cases.

A type I hypersensitivity response appears to play an important part in the pathogenesis of asthma. The recruitment of eosinophils into the mucosa results in the release of many inflammatory mediators. These include leukotrienes LTC4 and LTD4 which cause bronchoconstriction, and platelet activating factor (PAF) which results in long-lasting hyperresponsiveness of smooth muscle.

CASE 13

Mrs Nellie Fairburn is a 60-year-old woman who works at night as a cleaner. She has been involved in a warehouse fire in which she suffered severe burns to her legs. She had previously been fit and well and was on no medication prior to admission. She is nursed in a specialized burns unit and careful attention is given to her fluid balance. Twenty-four hours after admission she develops progressive respiratory distress. On examination, she is apyrexial, but tachypnoeic and centrally cyanosed with bilateral inspiratory crepitations.

Her condition deteriorates and she requires transfer to an intensive care unit where she is ventilated. Despite continuous positive, airway pressure ventilation and intensive support of cardiac and renal function she continued to deteriorate, eventually dying from multi-organ failure 10 days after admission.

Investigations	Results
Chest X-ray at 12 hours	normal
Chest X-ray at 48 hours	bilateral diffuse shadowing sparing apices and costophrenic angles
PaO_2 (on 60% O_2)	6.7 kPa

Questions

1 What is the diagnosis and why did this condition develop?
2 What is the pathophysiology of the condition?
3 What are the possible outcomes?

YOUR ANSWERS

1 Diagnosis and reasons for development

2 Pathophysiology of the condition

3 Possible outcomes

CASE 13 ANSWERS

pp. 173, 174

1 Diagnosis and reasons for development

This woman has developed adult respiratory distress syndrome (ARDS) which represents a reaction of the lung to a wide variety of insults. Precipitating factors in this case include the shock of severe burns and probable smoke inhalation.

2 Pathophysiology of condition

The initial insult produces damage to both alveolar-lining cells and capillary endothelial cells. In the acute phase of the disease, this causes necrosis of the alveolar epithelium and microthrombosis of the capillaries with neutrophil adherence and activation. Epithelial and endothelial cell damage results in interstitial oedema and exudation of blood, fibrin and fluid into the alveolar spaces with hyaline membrane formation. Later, in the organization phase, there is regeneration of type II pneumocytes and inflammation of the interstitium. Organization of the hyaline membranes results in interstitial fibrosis.

3 Possible outcomes

Despite intensive supportive therapy, in approximately 70% of cases death occurs in the acute phase. This is caused, as in this case, by the development of systemic inflammatory-response syndrome following the release of cytokines into the systemic circulation. This results in systemic endothelial activation with neutrophil activation, leading to multi-organ failure. Twenty percent of those who survive have some permanent lung dysfunction.

CASE 14

Mr Harvey Lopez is a 55-year-old man who has sold his business to concentrate on breeding racing pigeons, a consuming passion since the death of his son several years earlier in a tragic road traffic accident. He tells you that he has experienced recurrent episodes of feeling unwell, accompanied by a cough and severe shortness of breath lasting between 12 and 24 hours. Although he has a cough, he says that he does not bring anything up. In addition, over the previous year or so he has noticed a gradual loss of weight with episodic fevers and he reckons that he is not so fit, being unable to climb the stairs to his pigeon loft because of shortness of breath. He is a non-smoker and has been otherwise well on no medication. There is no family history of disease.

He has come during one of his attacks and on examination he is noted to have clubbing of the fingers, is pyrexial, centrally cyanosed and tachypnoeic. There are coarse expiratory crepitations heard throughout the lung fields.

Investigation	Result
White-cell count	Elevated with a neutrophilia
ESR	60 mm/hr
FEV1/FVC	Both reduced, ratio normal
Gas-transfer factor	Reduced
PaO_2	Reduced
$PaCO_2$	Reduced
Chest X-ray	Micronodular shadowing

Questions

1 What is your differential diagnosis?
2 What other investigations would you perform?
3 What pathological process is going on in the lungs?
4 What are its long-term complications?

YOUR ANSWERS

1 Differential diagnosis

2 Other investigations

3 Pathological process in lungs

4 Long-term complications

CASE 14 ANSWERS p. 177

1 Differential diagnosis

The results of the spirometry and blood-gas estimations indicate a restrictive ventilatory defect and the episodic nature suggests repeated exposure to a precipitating factor, most likely an allergen causing extrinsic allergic alveolitis. Specific questions should be asked about occupation, hobbies and pets.

2 Other investigations

Serological studies may show an increase in IgA and IgG in typical extrinsic allergic alveolitis. Specific antibodies may be detected by precipitin tests, but detection of precipitins neither indicate pathogenicity nor correlate with disease severity. They will exclude the diagnosis if negative. Detailed questioning revealed that the exacerbations of his symptoms would follow a few hours after cleaning out the pigeon loft. Precipitating antibodies against pigeon protein and droppings were subsequently detected.

3 Pathological process in lungs

Following acute exposure to the antigen there is a type III hypersensitivity response with formation of immune complexes, complement activation and inflammation. This results in dyspnoea, fever and cough 4–8 hours after exposure, typically resolving in 12–24 hours.

4 Long-term complications

With repeated antigen exposure, a type IV hypersensitivity response occurs with formation of small granulomata. This results in interstitial fibrosis with progressive cough and dyspnoea, eventually leading to end-stage honeycomb lung and cor pulmonale in about 5% of cases. The gradual weight loss, progressive reduction in exercise tolerance and digital clubbing suggest a degree of permanent impairment in this case.

CASE 15

Mr Arthur Forester is a 60-year-old man who had to give up his job as a naval-dockyard worker one year ago when the Government decided on a policy of running down the navy. He has been depressed since being made unemployed and now says that he has developed a troublesome cough, with breathlessness on exertion. He also says that he has lost weight. He has no significant past medical history and is on no medication. He stopped smoking 20 years ago. He has a dog but no other pets.

On examination, he has clubbing of the fingers and is tachypnoeic at rest. He is not clinically cyanosed. His JVP is elevated, he has a right parasternal heave, mild hepatomegaly and bilateral ankle oedema. Bilateral end-inspiratory crepitations can be heard on auscultation of the chest.

Treatment with corticosteroids was commenced but with little effect and he has continued to show progressive deterioration in respiratory and cardiac function.

Investigation	Result
FBC	Normal
FEV1/FVC	Ratio slightly increased, both reduced
Gas-transfer factor	Reduced
Chest X-ray	Linear basal shadowing, pleural plaques
PaO$_2$	10.2 kPa
ECG	Right-ventricular hypertrophy
Urea and electrolytes	Normal

Questions

1 What pathological process is going on in the lungs?
2 What aetiological factor is suggested?
3 What other respiratory complications are associated with this aetiology?
4 What are the histological features seen in the lungs and their pathogenesis?

YOUR ANSWERS

1 Pathological process in lungs

2 Suggested aetiological factor

3 Other respiratory complications associated with this aetiology

4 Histological features seen in the lungs and their pathogenesis

CASE 15 ANSWERS — pp. 173, 179

1 Pathological process in the lungs

The symptoms are those of gradually declining respiratory function and the investigations confirm mild hypoxaemia with a restrictive ventilatory defect. The chest X-ray features are in keeping with interstitial fibrosis. There are clinical features of right-heart failure and pulmonary hypertension.

2 Aetiological factor suggested

Someone of this age who has worked in a dockyard for many years may well have been exposed to asbestos and therefore be suffering from asbestosis. A further indication that this is so in this case is the presence of pleural plaques on chest X-ray. The most likely diagnosis is asbestosis.

3 Other respiratory complcations associated with this aetiology

In addition to asbestosis and pleural plaques, asbestos exposure is also associated with the development of:

- Pleural effusions
- Diffuse pleural fibrous thickening
- Development of malignant mesothelioma
- Asbestosis, which requires a prolonged and heavy exposure to asbestos, may be complicated by the development of bronchial carcinoma. Smokers who are exposed to asbestos have a markedly increased risk of developing carcinoma.

4 Histological features seen in lungs and their pathogenesis

The lungs show interstitial fibrosis, initially maximal at the lung bases, but eventually resulting in a honeycomb lung. The fibrosis follows the release of cytokines and the stimulation of fibroblasts as a result of macrophage activation, and local inflammation in response to the inhalation of the toxic asbestos. Asbestos bodies (fibres of asbestos coated in protein) may be identified.

CASE 16

Mrs Joan Swales is a 62-year-old woman who is still active in the fashion industry. She repeatedly tells you that she was one of the first people to sell mini-skirts. She is worried and has come to hospital because of a two month history of cough, haemoptysis, malaise and weight loss. More recently, she has developed a hoarse voice and an odd tingling sensation down the inner aspect of her left arm. She had smoked 25 cigarettes a day for 30 years and also has a history of angina for which her family practitioner has prescribed glyceryl trinitrate as required. She gives no relevant family history of disease.

On examination, she appears very thin. She has left partial ptosis, enophthalmos and meiosis. There is reduced sensation in the T1 dermatome on the left, with wasting of the left intrinsic hand muscles. Chest examination reveals dullness to percussion and bronchial breathing in the left upper zone.

A diagnosis of bronchial carcinoma was made and further investigations performed.

Investigation	Result
White-cell count	Moderate neutrophilia
ESR	50 mm/hr
Haemoglobin	Slightly reduced
Serum calcium	Elevated
Chest X-ray	Irregular round shadow in left apex with hilar enlargement
Bilirubin	Elevated
Alkaline phosphatase	Elevated

Questions

1 What is the pathological basis for her symptoms and signs?
2 Why is the serum calcium raised?
3 What further investigations would you perform?
4 What treatment options are there?

CASE 16 ANSWERS pp. 181–185

1 Pathological basis of symptoms and signs

General malaise and weight loss are non-specific features of malignancy. The cough and signs of consolidation may be the result either of infection distal to an airway blocked by tumour or of lymph node metastases. The haemoptysis is likely to be the result of ulceration of tumour in a bronchus. The recent hoarseness suggests recurrent laryngeal nerve palsy secondary to hilar involvement, and the wasting of hand muscles and parasthesia suggest infiltration of the brachial plexus. Ptosis, enophthalmos and meiosis form Horner's syndrome (together with reduced sweating of the affected side of the face) which implies spread into the cervical sympathetic chain.

2 Reason why serum calcium is raised

This may be the result of either metastatic bone involvement or the production of a parathyroid hormone-like substance (most commonly by squamous-cell carcinoma).

3 Further investigations

A tissue diagnosis should be sought and may be obtained by examining sputum cytology, cytology of a pleural effusion (if present), percutaneous needle biopsy or by obtaining a biopsy for histological examination at bronchoscopy.

Further investigation should be aimed at determining the tumour stage, and may include CT scan or MRI to assess local spread and liver ultrasound to identify hepatic metastases.

4 Treatment options

In this case, extensive local spread and probable hepatic and bone metastases indicate an advanced-stage and inoperable tumour. Depending on the histological type, the tumour may show a response to chemotherapy and/or radiotherapy.

CASE 17

Julia Bligh is a 13-year-old only child, doted on by two very protective parents who accompany her. Her father is an insurance underwriter and her mother is a lawyer specializing in medical negligence cases. Julia initially presented at the age of 10 feeling very unwell, with cough productive of yellow sputum, and shortness of breath. She has had many episodes of chest infections throughout childhood which were treated by her family practitioner. On examination, her height and weight are well below normal for her age. She has early clubbing of her fingers, and is pyrexial and tachypnoeic. Chest examination reveals signs of consolidation in the left lung base.

A diagnosis of cystic fibrosis with bronchiectasis is made. The chest infection is treated with appropriate antibiotics and physiotherapy. She recovers from this episode but continues to suffer from recurrent chest infections. She has recently developed glucose intolerance.

Investigation	Result
White-cell count	Elevated with neutrophilia
Haemoglobin	Normal
ESR	70 mm/hr
Urea and electrolytes	Normal
Chest X-ray	Left-basal shadowing with dilated airways
Blood culture	*Pseudomonas aeruginosa*
Sweat sodium chloride concentration	Elevated

Questions

1 How is this disease inherited?
2 What is its pathogenesis?
3 How does this affect the lung?
4 Why does bronchiectasis develop?

YOUR ANSWERS

1 Inheritance

2 Pathogenesis

3 Lung pathology

4 Pathogenesis of bronchiectasis

CASE 17 ANSWERS

pp. 191, 192, 270

1 Inheritance

Cystic fibrosis is an autosomal recessive disorder with 1 in 25 adults being heterozygous carriers of the CF gene which is located on the long arm of chromosome 7.

2 Pathogenesis

The CF gene encodes the cystic-fibrosis transmembrane-conductance regulator (CFTR). Absence or abnormal function of this protein prevents normal opening of chloride channels in response to raised cAMP. Thus, stimulated chloride secretion cannot occur and cells fail to secrete water and sodium resulting in extremely viscid mucus. A similar mechanism operates in the pancreas, again resulting in thick, viscid secretion. In the skin, defective active chloride reabsorption in the sweat gland ducts results in an abnormally high sweat-chloride concentration.

3 Lung's pathology

In the lung, obstruction and stagnation of secretions predisposes to recurrent infection. Trapping of air behind mucus plugs causes hyperinflation with an increased risk of developing a pneumothorax. Pulmonary hypertension and cor pulmonale eventually follow hypoxia, scarring and destruction of the pulmonary vascular bed.

4 Pathogenesis of bronchiectasis

This is abnormal dilatation of main bronchi and was identified on the chest X-ray in this case. In cystic fibrosis, both main pathogenic factors are present; the increased mucus viscosity interferes with drainage of secretions and recurrent infections weaken the bronchial walls.

CASE 18

Mr Bernard Briggs is a 58-year-old man who runs a shop selling spare parts for motor cycles. He can barely speak becase he is so short of breath. He tells you that he has always had a bad chest, coughing every day and producing copious green sputum. He also gets breathlessness on exertion. Over the past three days, his chest has become so much worse that he can barely move. He had smoked 30 cigarettes a day for over 40 years (60 pack-years) and also said that he occasionally developed chest pain on exertion which, to you, sounds like angina. He had only recently been prescribed a course of antibiotics but has been on no other medication. He has no significant family history of disease.

On examination, he is centrally cyanosed and pyrexial. He has a bounding pulse and shows peripheral vasodilatation. His JVP is elevated, and he has pitting ankle oedema and mild hepatomegaly. Examination of his chest reveals a right parasternal heave, coarse expiratory crepitations at the left base and expiratory wheeze.

Treatment with β-agonists results in an immediate slight improvement in the PEFR and, with appropriate antibiotics and physiotherapy, he gradually improves but remains breathless on exertion and continues to produce sputum on most days.

Investigation	Result
Full blood count	Elevated packed-cell volume
PaO_2	7.8 kPa
$PaCO_2$	7.2 KPa
PEFR	Low
FEV1/FVC	Ratio reduced
Chest X-ray	Overinflation with low, flat diaphragm and patchy, left-basal shadowing
ECG	Right-ventricular hypertrophy

Questions

1 What is the most likely diagnosis and what do the results of the investigations indicate?
2 What is the pathogenesis of his chest problem and what is the pathology in the bronchi?
3 What are the main risk factors for developing this disease?

YOUR ANSWERS

1 Diagnosis and results

2 Pathogenesis and pathology in bronchi

3 Risk factors

CASE 18 ANSWERS   pp. 159, 160, 172, 173

1 Diagnosis and results

The features are those an infective exacerbation of chronic obstructive pulmonary disease with symptoms of chronic bronchitis ('cough productive of sputum on most days for three months of the year for at least two consecutive years'). Some reversibility of the airways obstruction is indicated by the immediate partial response to β-agonists. The blood-gas analysis indicates a type II respiratory failure. The vasodilatation and bounding pulse are clinical features suggesting hypercapnia. The clinical features of right-heart failure and right-ventricular hypertrophy on ECG suggest pulmonary hypertension and the development of cor pulmonale.

A raised packed-cell volume suggests secondary polycythaemia following increased production of erythropoeitin in response to chronic hypoxaemia.

2 Pathogenesis and pathology in bronchi

The airways show mucus plugging and hyperplasia of mucin-secreting glands in their walls. There will be inflammaory changes due to the respiratory tract infection. Hypersecretion of mucus causes mucus plugging and obstruction of the bronchial lumen leading to alveolar hypoventilation, hypoxaemia and hypercapnia. Hypoxic pulmonary vasoconstriction may cause pulmonary hypertension and, eventually, cor pulmonale.

3 Risk factors

The main risk factors are a long history of smoking and poorly controlled asthma in childhood. Episodes of infection, as in this case, cause an acute decline in lung function and may precipitate an acute deterioration of chronic cor pulmonale.

CASE 19

Ms Alex Conaty is a 25-year-old musician on tour with a progressive jazz-saxophone quartet and is upset because she has been finding it difficult to play her instrument. She tells you that things started to go wrong after she developed 'big red gnat bites' on her shins and thighs which had appeared in crops over the previous two years. She also complains of bilateral knee- and ankle-joint pains. The thing that has finally brought her to see you is that she has been slowly getting more and more breathless, with a dry cough. She has no significant past history or family history of disease and is on no medication. She is a non-smoker.

On examination, red skin nodules up to 5 cm across are confirmed on her shins and she had a low-grade pyrexia. Finger clubbing is not present and there are no other findings of note.

A provisional diagnosis is made and following further investigation she is started on corticosteroid therapy which results in marked clinical improvement, with a fall in serum angiotensin-converting enzyme.

Questions

1 What is the most likely diagnosis and what is its cause?
2 What is the characteristic histological appearance?
3 What other manifestations may be seen in this condition?

YOUR ANSWERS

1 Diagnosis and cause

2 Histological appearance

3 Other manifestations

CASE 19 ANSWERS

pp. 180, 503

1 Diagnosis and cause

The most likely diagnosis is sarcoidosis associated with the skin rash of erythema nodosum. Although there are many causes of erythema nodosum, arthropathy, hilar lymphadenopathy and pulmonary infiltrates with a restrictive ventilatory defect, the combination of these features is highly suggestive of sarcoid.

2 Histological appearance

This is a granulomatous disease of unknown aetiology. Granulomas develop in many tissues, particularly lungs and lymph nodes. Within the lungs, interstitial infiltration leads to interstitial fibrosis. The finding of granulomas in the lung is further confirmation of the nature of the disease.

3 Other manifestations

This is a multisystem disease with granulomatous infiltrates that also commonly affects peripheral lymph nodes, the eyes, skin, spleen and salivary glands with less common involvement of the central nervous system and bones. Many patients, however, are asymptomatic, coming to light due to an abnormal chest radiograph. Main manifestations are combinations of:

- Lymphadenopathy.
- Lung disease.
- Iritis.
- Skin rash (erythema nodosum, lupus pernio).
- Hypercalcaemia.
- Peripheral neuropathy, cranial neuropathy, meningitis.
- Myopathy.
- Cardiomyopathy.

3

ORAL, EAR, NOSE AND THROAT PATHOLOGY

CASE 20

Mr Wayne Robinson, aged 19, a homeless vagrant, is seen in the Emergency Department in a drunken state. He is bleeding from the mouth. On examination, there is acute, sloughing ulceration of the gums surrounded by inflamed red mucosa, with many areas of bleeding. The breath is foul and the teeth are dirty. A smear from the ulcerated areas shows numerous fusiform and spirochaetal organisms.

QUESTIONS

1 What is the diagnosis?
2 What are the predisposing factors?
3 What are the organisms?
4 What are the long-term complications?

YOUR ANSWERS

1 Diagnosis

2 Predisposing factors

3 Organisms

4 Long-term complications

CASE 21

Mr Arnold Rimber, aged 72, is a retired bank clerk and is referred by his dentist because of an area of white thickening of the buccal mucosa. On examination, there is an ill-defined thick white patch on the buccal mucosa on the left. The lesion was biopsied.

QUESTIONS

1 What are the most likely causes?
2 Why was it considered important to biopsy the lesion?

YOUR ANSWERS

1 Likely causes

2 Reason for biopsy

CASE 20 ANSWERS p. 194

1 Diagnosis
Acute necrotising ulcerative gingivitis.

2 Predisposing factors
The disease is most common when there has been poor dental hygiene; it is usually seen in young males.

3 Organisms
The organisms are *Fusobacterium* and various types of *Borrelia*. These organisms are present in vast numbers in the necrotic slough in the ulcerated areas and between the teeth, and are considered to be the organisms responsible for the ulcerative gingivitis.

4 Long-term complications
In children in the Third World, acute ulcerative gingivitis may proceed to 'cancrum oris' – a severe oral infection that may destroy large areas of the lips and face. In young adults, however, the disease responds rapidly to oral metronidazole and rarely recurs, particularly if care is taken to remove plaque and calculus from around the teeth.

CASE 21 ANSWERS p. 196

1 Likely causes
The most likely diagnosis in a man of this age is frictional keratosis (due to chronic friction from ill-fitting dentures) or smoker's keratosis (seen in smokers, particularly pipe smokers). Other causes such as lichen planus and thrush (due to *Candida* infection) are less likely in a man of this age.

2 Reason for biopsy
Biopsy was undertaken to exclude the presence of dysplasia in the squamous epithelium. Early *in situ* or invasive squamous carcinomas in the mouth may present with a persistent white patch of thickening of the mucosa.

CASE 22

Mr Paulus Jurgens, aged 74, a retired tug pilot from the port of Liverpool, is seen because of an area of white thickening on the lateral border of the anterior third of his tongue. He had been aware of a slowly enlarging thick white patch for many months but it had caused him no concern until a small, slightly painful ulcer had developed in the centre of the patch. The lesion is biopsied to confirm the clinical diagnosis before curative treatment was initiated.

Questions

1 What is the most likely clinical diagnosis?
2 If the biopsy confirms the clinical diagnosis, what is the most frequent and effective form of treatment?
3 What is the commonest site for spread of the lesion?

YOUR ANSWERS

1 Diagnosis

2 Treatment

3 Site for spread

CASE 23

Mrs Consuela Lombardo, once famous as a stage star and still in demand for chat shows, is now aged 57. She has come somewhat unwillingly to hospital because of a smooth, enlarging mass at the angle of the jaw on the left side. She says it has been present for some years, had given her no trouble but had slowly enlarged and was now becoming disfiguring. Her anxious daughter feared cancer, and the lump could no longer be disguised by cosmetics. On examination, the mass appears to be in the parotid gland, is firm and rubbery, with a smooth well-circumscribed outline, and is non-tender.

Questions

1 What is the differential diagnosis?
2 What precautions must be taken during surgery and why?

YOUR ANSWERS

1 Diagnosis

2 Surgical care

CASE 22 ANSWERS   p. 197

1 Diagnosis
Invasive squamous carcinoma of the tongue, arising in an area of carcinoma *in situ*.

2 Treatment
Wide, local excision of the tumour, often a hemiglossectomy; these tumours often infiltrate deeply and extensively despite being apparently small on the surface. Surgical excision of the primary tumour may be combined with block dissection of the neck on the same side to include the local and regional lymph nodes, including those in the jugular chain.

3 Site for spread
Regional lymph nodes in the neck – hence the importance of a block dissection in advanced cases.

CASE 23 ANSWERS   p. 198

1 Diagnosis
The most likely diagnosis is pleomorphic salivary adenoma, a benign tumour of the salivary gland. Adenolymphoma, another benign tumour, is possible but less likely. Adenoid cystic carcinoma, the most common malignant tumour of salivary tissue, is much less likely, bearing in mind the long history, slow growth, and smooth, well-defined outline. However, certain diagnosis can only be made by excision biopsy, although fine needle aspiration cytology may be used to exclude malignancy before curative surgery.

2 Surgical care
Benign, pleomorphic salivary adenoma can recur if any small fragments are left behind at surgery. It is therefore advisable to remove the tumour with a safe margin of normal parotid tissue; this is sometimes a problem because of the proximity of the facial nerve which runs between the deep and superficial parts of the parotid gland.

CASE 24

Elizabeth Roystone, a 23-year-old audio-typist, has had to take considerable time off work because of deafness in her right ear associated with chronic earache and intermittent but persistent discharge of purulent fluid. On examination, she is found to have a perforation of the eardrum in the attico-antral region through which an irregular white mass is protruding.

Questions

1 What is the most likely explanation for her earache, deafness and discharge?
2 What is the likely cause for the white material protruding through the atticoantral perforation of the eardrum?
3 What are the major complications of this condition?

YOUR ANSWERS

1 Diagnosis

2 Nature of white material

3 Complications

CASE 25

Estelle Pentouselle, a 42-year-old Parisian chanteuse is unable to fulfil her professional obligations in the 4ième arrondissement because of increasing hoarseness of voice which had been present for many months. Initially, the symptom gave her voice a smoky, throaty timbre that was much appreciated by her audience, but the symptoms have worsened so that she is scarcely capable of singing at all. She had reduced her smoking from 30 Gauloises per day to less than five, but there had been little or no improvement.

Questions

1 What is the diagnosis?
2 What would her larynx look like on direct laryngoscopy and what is the nature of the lesions?

YOUR ANSWERS

1 Diagnosis

2 Appearance and nature

CASE 24 ANSWERS

pp. 209, 210

1 Diagnosis

The symptoms are those of chronic suppurative otitis media, which is usually associated with perforation of the eardrum, either tubotympanic (in the centre of the eardrum) or attico-antral (with the perforation in the attic region).

2 Nature of white material

The white material is almost certainly masses of packed keratin arising from a cholesteatoma in the epitympanic recess (the attic) and the mastoid antrum. A cholesteatoma is an enlarging cystic mass lined by stratified squamous epithelium which produces large amounts of white keratin, resembling an epidermoid cyst. The constant production of keratin leads to progressive enlargement of the cyst, eventually eroding structures in the ear cavity, such as the labyrinth, facial nerve and mastoid air cells.

3 Complications

The major complication of cholesteatoma is irreversible deafness due to destruction of ear structures by the enlarging keratin-containing lesion. Large lesions may erode the skull through the base of the middle cranial fossa, and bacterial super-infection of the cholesteatoma contents can lead to brain abscess and meningitis.

CASE 25 ANSWERS

p. 214

1 Diagnosis

She almost certainly has singer's nodules.

2 Appearance and nature

Singer's nodules appear as smooth, round nodules on the true cord located at the junction between the anterior third and posterior two-thirds. They are foci of submucosal fibrosis. Because of her smoking habits, she may also have smoker's keratosis in which the true cords are thickened by an increase in thickness of squamous epithelium and the overlying keratin layer.

CASE 26

Mr Eli Rathbone, aged 68, is a retired pigman who lives on the farm which is now run by his son. He has been a heavy smoker of hand-rolled cigarettes for over 50 years, and has had a hoarse voice for as long as he can remember. He attends hospital complaining of complete loss of voice present for about one month. On laryngoscopy, the left vocal cord is completely replaced by a large white friable mass which extends to the anterior commissure. The right vocal cord is thickened and irregular.

Questions

1 What is wrong with his left vocal cord?
2 What is wrong with his right vocal cord?
3 What is the most likely sequence of events?
4 What will happen in the future if the lesion is not successfully treated?

YOUR ANSWERS

1 Left-cord abnormality

2 Right-cord abnormality

3 Sequence of events

4 Outcome with treatment

CASE 26 ANSWERS

p. 214

1 Left-cord abnormality

The left cord has developed an invasive squamous carcinoma.

2 Right-cord abnormality

The right vocal cord will almost certainly show a mixture of smoker's keratosis (in which the squamous epithelium is thickened, covered by a thick layer of keratin, and may show dysplastic changes), together with carcinoma *in situ* (in which the dysplastic changes in the squamous epithelial cells are much more severe).

3 Sequence of events

The likely sequence of events is:
- Heavy smoking.
- Smoker's keratosis of the larynx.
- Carcinoma *in situ*.
- Invasive squamous carcinoma.

4 Outcome without treatment

Although the invasive tumour appears to be confined to the true cord (i.e. it is 'glottic') the prognosis may be poor because it has spread to the anterior commissure where there are abundant lymphatics and vessels; thus, the opportunity for metastatic spread to the lymph nodes in the neck is greatly increased.

4

ALIMENTARY SYSTEM

CASE 27

Ms Odette Forbes is a 25-year-old talented ballet dancer who is at present studying a major role in a modern work. She presents with intermittent dull abdominal pain. She tells you that during the previous six months she had had several episodes of diarrhoea, sometimes associated with passage of fresh red blood and mucus. This has, understandably, interfered with her work. She had also lost some weight and had recently developed joint pains.

On abdominal examination, there is much voluntary guarding with a suggestion of tenderness in the left iliac fossa. No lesions are palpated on rectal examination but an anal fissure and skin tags are noticed.

Barium enema is performed which showed deep ulcers in the region of the sigmoid colon with tracking along the submucosa. A barium meal and follow through demonstrate a long irregular stricture in the terminal ileum.

On colonoscopy, the rectum appears normal, but there are intermittent foci of congestion and irregularity of the mucosa with a cobblestone appearance. The examination is extended round to the terminal ileum and multiple biopsies are taken.

Investigation	Result
Colonoscopic biopsies	There are patchy acute and chronic inflammatory cells extending into the submucosa. Both the terminal ileal and caecal biopsies show several non-caseating epithelioid-cell granulomas
Blood count and film	Mild iron-deficiency anaemia
Ferritin and B_{12}	Low ferritin and low normal B_{12}
Liver-function tests	Low normal albumin
ESR	Mildly raised

Questions

1 What differential diagnoses should be considered with this presentation?
2 In view of the radiological, colonoscopic and biopsy findings, what is the final diagnosis?
3 What other disease processes of the small and large intestine show granulomas on histology?
4 What are the main non-gastrointestinal manifestations of chronic inflammatory bowel disease?

YOUR ANSWERS

1 Differential diagnoses considered with this presentation

2 Final diagnosis

3 Granulomas in other disease processes of the intestine

4 Main non-gastrointestinal manifestations of chronic inflammatory bowel disease

CASE 27 ANSWERS   pp. 228-230

1 Differential diagnoses considered with this presentation

Inflammatory bowel disease is the likely diagnosis; in view of the presence of anal disease, Crohn's disease is much more likely than ulcerative colitis. The symptoms of infective-type colitis may mimic inflammatory bowel disease but, in that situation, the history is usually days or weeks rather than months.

2 Final diagnosis

These features are entirely consistent with Crohn's disease. Terminal ileal involvement and patchy inflammation with granulomas are typical.

3 Granulomas in other disease processes of the intestine

Tuberculosis, some rarer infections and, rarely, foreign-body reaction.

4 Main non-gastrointestinal manifestations of inflammatory bowel disease

These include enteropathic arthritis, ankylosing spondylitis, iritis, aphthous stomatitis, sclerosing cholangitis, erythema nodosum and pyoderma gangrenosum.

CASE 28

Mr Josh Dawson is a 45-year-old man who works occasionally as a dishwasher, but who mainly keeps himself on social security payments. He has been brought to hospital by ambulance having collapsed in the street, vomiting blood. He tells you that he has had recurrent pains in his stomach, on and off, for two years and points to his epigastrium. This occasionally wakes him at night. The pain is usually relieved by taking antacids or food. You think he probably has an ulcer in the upper GI tract.

Endoscopy shows a gastric ulcer on the lesser curve of stomach, at the junction of the body and antrum. Bleeding continues and partial gastrectomy is performed. Histology confirms a chronic gastric ulcer which had eroded an artery in its base.

Questions

1 What are the possible causes of this clinical presentation?
2 What are the predisposing factors to peptic gastric ulceration?
3 What are the complications of peptic ulceration?

YOUR ANSWERS

1 Possible causes of this presentation

2 Predisposing factors for ulcer formation

3 Complications of peptic gastric ulceration

CASE 29

Mr Gaston Lafayette is a 57-year-old restauranteur. He has presented with a history of a retrosternal burning sensation, particularly after large meals and often on retiring to bed at night. Treatment with antacids did little to relieve the discomfort. He is referred for endoscopy. This did not show a hiatus hernia but the lower oesophagus showed reddening from the level of the oesophago–gastric junction to a point 32 cm from the incisors. The proximal border of the reddened area was irregular. A biopsy was taken from the lower oesophagus which showed gastric and intestinal-type glandular mucosa.

Questions

1 What is the likely cause of the symptoms?
2 What is the final diagnosis?
3 What further information do you require from the biopsy report?

YOUR ANSWERS

1 Likely cause of the symptoms

2 Final diagnosis

3 Further information required from biopsy report

CASE 28 ANSWERS p. 223

1 Possible causes of this presentation?

Bleeding peptic ulcer, whether gastric or duodenal, is the most likely diagnosis.

Other possible causes of haematemesis include:

- Oesophageal varices – associated with features of portal hypertension.
- Mallory–Weiss tear – associated with violent vomiting, often alcohol induced.
- Gastric carcinoma – should be suspected in an older patient with a history of anorexia, easy satiety and loss of weight.

Rarer causes include:

- Acute gastric ulcer – aspirin or alcohol induced.
- Ulcerating oesophagitis.

2 Predisposing factors for ulcer formation

In the stomach, initial epithelial damage is caused by by *H. pylori* infection, non-steroidal anti-inflammatory drugs, and regurgitation of bile from the duodenum. Once epithelium is damaged, gastric acid perpetuates ulceration and leads to chronicity.

3 Complications of peptic gastric ulceration

Haemorrhage, chronicity, penetration, perforation, gastric-outlet obstruction due to fibrous scarring and stricture. Uncommonly, development of carcinoma.

CASE 29 ANSWERS pp. 218, 219

1 Likely cause of the symptoms

The symptoms ('heartburn') are suggestive of gastro–oesophageal reflux, with or without the presence of a hiatus hernia. Other important causes of retrosternal pain should not be overlooked, including cardiovascular causes, especially myocardial ischaemia, as well as other rarer causes including pneumothorax and musculoskeletal pain.

2 Final diagnosis

The endoscopic and biopsy appearances confirm a Barrett's oesophagus. This is a metaplastic process which develops due to persistent reflux of gastric contents into the oesophagus, the normal squamous mucosa being replaced by glandular mucosa of gastric or intestinal type.

3 Further information required from biopsy report

It is important to look for dysplastic change in the biopsy which may herald the development of adenocarcinoma.

CASE 30

Robert Gallie is a six-year-old-boy who has been taken to the family practitioner by his mother because he has been complaining of abdominal pain occurring after some meals. This has been getting increasingly frequent and it sounds, from his description, somewhat colicky in nature. You discover that he has always had very smelly, loose, pale, bulky stools, which his parents had put down to the fact that he liked milk. On examination he is pale, moderately underweight and of short stature. His abdomen is mildly distended.

Investigation	Result
Blood count and film	Mild macrocytic anaemia. Howell–Jolly bodies
Haematinics	Low vitamin B_{12}, folate low normal
Antigliadin antbody	Positive
Jejunal biopsy	Villous atrophy, increased intraepithelial and lamina propria lymphocytes

Questions

1 What are the important differential diagnoses on presentation?
2 What is the likely reason for the blood abnormalities?
3 What is the final diagnosis and management?

CASE 30 ANSWERS
pp. 226, 227

1 Important differential diagnoses on presentation

Coeliac disease is the most likely diagnosis. Parasitic infestation (e.g. Giardiasis) and pancreatic insufficiency (e.g. due to chronic pancreatitis or cystic fibrosis) may give rise to similar presentation but these are not supported by the results of investigations.

2 Reason for blood abnormalities

Malabsorbtion of vitamin B_{12} and folate from abnormal small-bowel mucosa.

3 Likely diagnosis and management

The most likely diagnosis is coeliac disease due to hypersensitivity to alpha gliadin, a component of gluten, leading to small intestinal villous atrophy. The final diagnosis of coeliac disease is confirmed by symptomatic resolution on a gluten-free diet, and symptomatic and histologic relapse on re-challenge. Such rigorous criteria are neccessary before confining a patient to a life-long gluten-free diet. Relapse of symptoms is usually due to inadequate dietary compliance, but the development of collagenous sprue (treatable with steroids) and small bowel lymphoma should be considered.

CASE 31

Mrs Wilma Witherspoon is a 72-year-old widow. Her husband had been a commercial pilot and had died three years earlier after a dementing illness. She has presented with intermittent episodes of vomiting, which has been accompanied by gradually increasing abdominal distension and discomfort. On examination her abdominen is distended and she is otherwise very thin. On abdominal percussion there is 'shifting dullness' indicating that excess peritoneal fluid is the cause of the distension. There is also an umbilical hernia.

Investigation	Result
Abdominal ultrasound	Ascites; left ovarian mass 13 cm in diameter; normal liver, spleen and kidneys
Paracentesis and cytology	Adenocarcinoma cells and psammoma bodies present

Questions

1 What are the important possible causes of ascites?
2 What is the diagnosis?
3 What is the cause of the vomiting?

CASE 32

Mr Fred Greengrass, a 67-year-old retired dairy farmer, has come to medical attention because he says he is having trouble with his guts. He has developed alternating diarrhoea and constipation for approximately six weeks. He also had intermittent abdominal pain but had lost no weight. He has become worried because he has noticed some blood mixed with his faeces. On examination, he is tender in his lower abdomen and there is the suggestion of a mass in the left iliac fossa. Proctoscopic examination showed first degree haemorrhoids but no other abnormality.

Investigation	Result
Blood count and film	Mild, hypochromic, microcytic anaemia
Barium enema	Multiple sigmoid diverticula with marked thickening of the bowel wall

Questions

1 What are the important differential diagnoses with this pattern of altered bowel habit?
2 What are the pathological features of diverticular disease?
3 What are the important complications of diverticular disease?
4 What is the reason for the blood abnormality?

CASE 31 ANSWERS p. 239

1 Causes of ascites

The main causes of ascites are tumours involving the peritoneal cavity, inflammation of the peritoneum, and increased transudation from vessels caused by increased pressure in the portal venous system. The main cause of the latter are cirrhosis of the liver, portral vein thrombosis or Budd–Chiari syndrome.

2 Diagnosis

Peritoneal infiltration by ovarian carcinoma. This type of carcinoma may have small calcified areas termed 'psammoma bodies' which can be recognised histologically.

3 Cause of the vomiting

The most likely cause of vomiting is small bowel obstruction due to peritoneal tumour infiltration and adhesions.

CASE 32 ANSWERS p. 236

1 Differential diagnoses

The main processes causing this pattern of altered bowel habit are diverticular disease, colorectal carcinoma and ischaemic colitis.

2 Pathological features of diverticular disease

Herniation of the mucosa of the colon through the muscularis propria to form out-pouches of the bowel lumen. There is thickening of the muscularis propria.

3 Complications of diverticular disease

Acute diverticulitis, haemorrhage, perforation (causing peritonitis or paracolic abscess), and fibrous scarring causing obstuction.

4 Blood abnormality

Iron-deficiency anaemia, most likely from blood loss associated with the bowel disease.

CASE 33

Miss Felicity Rush is the 68-year-old part-owner of an organic food cooperative. She presents with complaints that, despite a wholefood diet, she has been getting intermittent constipation. She also has lost some weight and has noticed that she has a swollen abdomen. She says that she has noticed no passage of blood with bowel motions. Reviewing her records you note that three years previously, during investigation for iron deficiency anaemia, she was found to have two polyps of the sigmoid colon; these were removed endoscopically and histology showed a tubular and a tubulovillous adenoma.

Colonoscoscopy is performed and gives good visualization of the colon round to the transverse colon only, and no lesions are seen. Double-contrast barium enema shows an irregular stricture with shouldered edges approximately 4 cm in length in the ascending colon. A tumour is diagnosed and surgery is advised.

The tumour is resected and is found to have invaded through the full thickness of the bowel wall but is completely excised. Three of 15 lymph nodes identified contained metastatic tumour.

Questions

1 What is the most likely diagnosis with this presentation?
2 What stage is this tumour and what is the prognosis for this patient?
3 What is the association between adenoma and carcinoma?
4 Where is metastatic spread most likely?

YOUR ANSWERS

1 Diagnosis

2 Stage of tumour and prognosis

3 Association between adenoma and carcinoma

4 Metastatic spread

CASE 33 ANSWERS pp. 231, 234

1 Diagnosis

The most likely diagnosis is colorectal adenocarcinoma.

2 Stage of tumour and prognosis

This is a Dukes C carcinoma (note: several local variants of this staging scheme are in use, so check which applies in your own centre). Tumours of the right colon tend to present later than those of the distal colon because the bowel contents are more fluid and so obstruction occurs later. There is about 30% five-year survival with this stage of disease.

3 Association between colonic adenoma and carcinoma

There is much evidence to suggest that most carcinomas of the colon arise in pre-existing adenomas (adenoma–cancer sequence). Patients with familial adenomatosis coli have a very high risk of developing colorectal carcinoma.

4 Metastatic spread

Colorectal adenocarcinomas mainly metastasise to lymph nodes and liver, less commonly developing other systemic metastases.

HEPATOBILIARY SYSTEM AND PANCREAS

CASE 34

Mr Kevin Millbank is a 29-year-old estate agent whose business has collapsed and who is now living rough. He presents because he has been feeling nauseous and generally unwell for three days. On examination, he has a mild pyrexia and is tender in the right upper quadrant of his abdomen. He has been drinking one or two bottles of spirits a day.

A diagnosis of alcoholic hepatitis is made. After a period of time in hospital during which time he is treated with vitamins, a needle biopsy of the liver is performed.

Questions

1 What pathological changes may alcohol produce in the liver?
2 What proportion of patients with chronic alcoholism develop cirrhosis?
3 How do you prepare a patient with liver disease for biopsy?

Investigation	Result
Full blood count	Mild macrocytosis
Serum bilirubin	Moderately elevated
Serum alanine transaminase	Greatly elevated
Serum aspartate transaminase	Greatly elevated
Serum alkaline transaminase	Mildly elevated
Urate	Raised
Serum albumin	Normal
APTT	Slightly prolonged
Hepatitis-B serology	Negative

YOUR ANSWERS

1 Pathological changes in the liver caused by alcohol

2 Proportion of chronic alcoholics developing cirrhosis

3 Preparation of patient for liver biopsy

CASE 34 ANSWERS   p. 257

1 Pathological changes in the liver caused by alcohol?
Alcohol is an hepatotoxin, and liver damage is related to daily alcohol intake. Maximum recommended daily intakes have been defined when the risk of liver damage is thought to be small (50–60 g per day in men and 30–40 g per day in women). Women are more prone to alcohol-induced liver damage than men.

There are three patterns of alcoholic liver damage:
- **Fatty liver** – accumulation of fat in hepatocytes which is reversible with abstinence.
- **Acute alcoholic hepatitis** – ingestion of large amounts of alcohol causes a true hepatitis with focal necrosis of liver cells. If a patient with alcoholic hepatitis abstains, then this resolves without harm. With continued ingestion of alcohol, fibrosis develops around central veins and also in response to continued hepatocyte necrosis.
- **Alcoholic cirrhosis**.

2 Proportion of chronic alcoholics developing cirrhosis?
Cirrhosis develops in less than 10% of patients suffering from chronic alcoholism. It may develop after episodes of acute alcoholic hepatitis or may be insidious in its onset and only present as end-stage liver disease.

3 Preparation of the patient for liver biopsy
(i) Obtain informed consent.
(ii) Check prothrombin time, haemoglobin concentration and platelet count.
(iii) If all are normal, cross match two units of blood and proceed with biopsy.
(iv) If prothrombin time is abnormal and patient is not jaundiced, give vitamin K until prothrombin time < 1.3, then proceed.
(v) If prothrombin time is abnormal and patient is jaundiced, give slow intravenous vitamin K until prothrombin time is < 1.3, then proceed.
(vi) If the prothrombin time remains prolonged despite vitamin K, and the biopsy is essential, carry out biopsy whilst giving fresh frozen plasma. Check prothrombin time before and after the biopsy.

CASE 35

Mr Joseph Zamway is a 55-year-old pensions-fund manager for a large national publishing concern. He has been admitted to hospital for investigation of increasing cardiac failure. Examination reveals that he has an enlarged liver. It is noticed that his skin is a uniform dark colour.

A diagnosis of haemochromatosis is made.

Questions
1 What is the inheritance of this disorder?
2 What pathology occurs in the liver?
3 What is the reason for abnormal glucose tolerance?
4 After correctly diagnosing and treating Mr Zamway, what else must be done?

Investigation	Result
Urine	Glycosuria
Blood glucose	Abnormally high
Serum iron	Elevated
Serum ferritin	Greatly elevated
Transferrin saturation	Greatly elevated
Liver biopsy	Hepatocytes and Kupffer cells packed with haemosiderin seen with Perls' stain

YOUR ANSWERS

1 Inheritance

2 Pathology in liver

3 Abnormal glucose tolerance

4 What else must be done?

CASE 35 ANSWERS   p. 258

1 Inheritance
This is an autosomal recessive disorder.

2 Pathology in liver
Accumulation of iron in the liver causes death of hepatocytes (possibly from the generation of free radicals) and leads to cirrhosis. There is a predisposition for development of primary hepatocellular carcinoma.

3 Abnormal glucose tolerance
Accumulation of iron in the pancreatic islets causes diabetes mellitus, while accumulation in the cardiac muscle causes a cardiomyopathy with heart failure.

4 What else must be done?
His first degree relatives must be screened by blood tests to check their ferritin and transferrin saturation. If raised, the diagnosis must be confirmed by liver biopsy.

CASE 36

Mr Roger Flambards is a 60-year-old retired stockbroker. He is seen because he has bilateral parotid enlargement, a right Dupuytren's contracture, and has developed increasing abdominal swelling. On examination it is apparent that the cause of his abdominal swelling is ascites. He also has spider naevi, mild ankle oedema, splenomegaly, and a firm, slightly enlarged liver. Further investigations are performed.

After correction of his blood clotting abnormality, a liver biopsy is performed which shows established cirrhosis with features consistent with an alcoholic causation.

Investigation	Result
Full blood count	Macrocytosis (round)
Serum bilirubin	Moderately elevated
Serum alanine transaminase	Moderately elevated
Serum aspartate transaminase	Moderately elevated
Serum alkaline phosphatase	Mildly elevated
Serum albumin	Reduced
APTT	Greatly prolonged
Hepatitis-B serology	Negative
Blood ethanol (10.30am)	80 mg/dl

Questions

1 What are the pathological features seen in the liver in cirrhosis?
2 What histological features would have been seen to suggest an alcoholic causation?
3 What are the complications of cirrhosis?

YOUR ANSWERS

1 Pathological features of cirrhosis

2 Histological features suggesting an alcoholic causation

3 Complications of cirrhosis

CASE 36 ANSWERS

pp. 259, 260

1 Pathological features of cirrhosis

In cirrhosis, the normal architecture of the liver is diffusely replaced by nodules of regenerated liver cells separated by bands of collagenous fibrosis. It is an irreversible form of chronic liver disease which is the end stage of many processes. It has three common factors:

- Long-standing destruction of liver cells.
- Associated inflammation that stimulates fibrosis.
- Regeneration of hepatocytes to cause nodules.

2 Histological features suggesting an alcoholic causation

Prominent fatty change and the presence of Mallory's hyaline are suggestive of alcoholic liver damage.

3 Complications of cirrhosis

The main consequences of cirrhosis are:

- Reduced hepatocyte function – decreased synthesis of proteins, failure of detoxification.
- Disturbance of blood flow through the liver causing portal hypertension with all its attendant complications, particularly ascites and oesophageal varices.
- Reduced immune competence and increased susceptibility to infection.
- Increased risk of development of hepatocellular carcinoma.
- Increased risk of development of portal vein thrombosis.

CASE 37

Mrs Mary Maggs is a 52-year-old bakery assistant. She has come to her family doctor because of increasingly troublesome generalized itching. On examination, she is not jaundiced and there are no stigmata of chronic liver disease. Investigations are performed.

A diagnosis of primary biliary cirrhosis is made and she is referred to a liver disease specialist for a liver biopsy to assess the stage of disease and she is treated with ursodeoxycholic acid.

Investigation	Result
Full blood count and ESR	Normal
Blood sugar	Normal
Alkaline phosphatase	Very high
Bilirubin	Moderately elevated
AST and ALT	Mildly elevated
Albumin	Normal
Prothrombin time	Mildly prolonged
Immunology	Antimitochondrial auto-antibodies (titre >1:40) elevated levels of serum IgM

Questions

1 What are the histological changes seen in primary biliary cirrhosis (PBC)?
2 What is thought to be the pathogenesis of the disease?
3 What is the natural history of this disease?

CASE 37 ANSWERS p. 262

1 Histological changes in PBC

Liver biopsy is performed to evaluate the stage of the disease. Biopsy of liver in early disease reveals obliteration of bile ducts in portal tracts associated with small granulomas. There is infiltration of portal tracts by lymphoid cells with destruction of adjacent hepatocytes in a manner similar to piecemeal necrosis. As disease progresses, there is fibrosis and proliferation of small bile ducts at the periphery of the portal tracts. In the final stages of disease, there is development of cirrhosis.

2 Pathogenesis of PBC

PBC is ten times more common in women than men and is one of the common causes of chronic liver disease and cirrhosis in women over the age of 50. Although immune phenomena are involved in disease, the aetiology of primary biliary cirrhosis is uncertain.

3 Natural history of PBC

There is gradual progression of disease over about 10 years. Treatment with ursodeoxycholic acid delays progression, but liver transplantation is often necessary.

CASE 38

Mr Eric Gribble is an unemployed 49-year-old security guard, recently dismissed after several prisoners escaped from his custody. His personal circumstances had not improved and he had been recently separated from his wife because of several episodes of domestic violence. He is admitted as an emergency to hospital accompanied by a friend. The two of them had been having a drinking session which had been going on for about five days. His friend had called around to go out when he had found Eric collapsed in the kitchen hunched forward over a chair with severe abdominal pain. An ambulance had been called.

On examination, he is shocked and has severe abdominal tenderness. After an intravenous line and a nasogastric tube are inserted, investigations are performed.

A diagnosis of acute pancreatitis is made.

Questions

1 What are the main causes of acute pancreatitis?
2 What is the pathogenesis of acute pancreatitis?
3 What are complications of acute pancreatitis?

Investigation	Result
Full blood count and ESR	Neutrophil leukocytosis
Serum amylase	Greatly elevated
Serum albumin	Moderately reduced
Serum calcium	Reduced
Bilirubin	Mildly elevated
Serum alanine transaminase	Mildly elevated
Serum aspartate transaminase	Mildly elevated
Serum alkaline phosphatase	Mildly elevated
Abdominal X-ray	No free air seen beneath diaphragm

YOUR ANSWERS

1 Causes of acute pancreatitis

2 Pathogenesis of acute pancreatitis

3 Complications of acute pancreatitis

CASE 38 ANSWERS
p. 269

1 Causes of acute pancreatitis
Mechanical obstruction of pancreatic ducts:
- Gallstones.
- Trauma.
- Post-operative.

Metabolic/toxic causes:
- Alcohol.
- Drugs (e.g. thiazide diuretics, azathioprine).
- Hypercalcaemia.
- Hypertriglyceridaemia.

Vascular/poor perfusion:
- Atherosclerosis.
- Hypothermia.

Infections:
- Mumps.

2 Pathogenesis of acute pancreatitis
Severe acute inflammation and necrosis of the pancreas is caused by the liberation of the powerful digestive enzymes; this results in extensive enzyme-mediated local tissue necrosis, particularly fat necrosis. Three patterns of pancreatic necrosis have been defined:

- **Periductal necrosis –** necrosis takes place in acinar cells adjacent to ducts. This form is seen in conditions caused by duct obstruction, particularly associated with gallstones, and alcohol.
- **Perilobular necrosis –** necrosis takes place in the periphery of lobules. The pathogenesis is poor vascular perfusion of this zone leading to acinar necrosis. This pattern is seen in shock and hypothermia.
- **Panlobular necrosis –** necrosis is found affecting all portion so the pancreatic lobule. This may be due to spread from initial periductal or perilobular necrosis or may be panlobular from the start.

3 Complications of acute pancreatitis
Clinically, most patients with acute pancreatitis recover. A complication of the development of acute pancreatitis is the conversion of the necrotic pancreas into a cyst filled with sero–sanguinous fluid termed a 'pancreatic pseudocyst'.

In severe disease, chemical peritonitis and shock may develop and can be fatal. This may predispose to adult respiratory distress syndrome.

6

LYMPHOID AND HAEMOPOEITIC SYSTEM

CASE 39

Mr Bill Sykes is a 72-year-old retired steel erector. He has undergone biopsy of one of a group of enlarged cervical lymph nodes which have been present for about six weeks. You phone the laboratory for a report and the pathologist dictates a preliminary report as follows:
- Macroscopic findings: lymph node, 2 cm in maximum extent with a focally yellow cut surface.
- Microscopic findings: the lymph node contains multiple well-formed granulomata.

Questions

1 From the preliminary report, what is the differential diagnosis?
2 What other investigations would be appropriate?
3 Describe a typical granuloma and the mechanisms important in its formation.

YOUR ANSWERS

l Casuses of granulomatous inflammation within lymph nodes

2 Other investigations

3 Description of granuloma

CASE 40

Ms Natalia Martin is a 26-year-old hospital kitchen worker. As part of her occupational health surveillance she has a chest X-ray. This is reported as showing mediastinal lymphadenopathy. When she is questioned further she says that she has had occasional bouts of fever and night sweats and has lost about one stone in weight over the preceding six months. A thorough physical examination reveals cervical lymphadenopathy and a node is removed for histological assessment. The report confirms the presence of Hodgkin's disease (HD).

Questions

1 What is necessary for the histological diagnosis of Hodgkin's disease and how are the different forms of the disease classified?
2 What is the Ann Arbor Staging System and what are the implications for therapy?
3 What factors are important in the prognosis of HD?

YOUR ANSWERS

l Diagnosis of Hodgkin's disease

2 Ann Arbor Staging System

3 Prognosis

CASE 39 ANSWERS   pp. 76, 273

1 Causes of granulomatous inflammation within lymph nodes
- Mycobacterial infection.
- Sarcoidosis.
- Cat-scratch disease.
- Toxoplasmosis.
- Fungal infection (e.g. *Histoplasma*).
- Other bacteria (e.g. *Yersinia, Brucella*).
- Crohn's disease.
- Rarer causes (e.g. reaction to Hodgkin's Disease).

2 Other investigations
Part of the lymph node should have been sent for culture, including for TB. Mycobacterial organisms may take 4–6 weeks to grow. Other investigations (which may already have been done) should include a chest X-ray, sputum microscopy and culture and a Mantoux test. Staining of the node for acid-fast bacilli as well as fungi should be performed.

3 Description of granuloma
A granuloma is a collection of histiocytes, epithelioid macrophages and possibly giant cells with or without a mantle of lymphocytes. It is a manifestation of cell-mediated immunity and a Type IV hypersensitivity response.

CASE 40 ANSWERS   pp. 275, 277

1 Diagnosis of Hodgkin's disease
The diagnosis of HD requires the presence of the neoplastic Reed–Sternberg (RS) cells (or variants thereof) within an appropriate cellular background. Four main types are described in the Rye classification. The difference between the types is in the vigour of the host response.
- In lymphocyte-predominant HD the node is replaced by reactive lymphoid cells with occasional RS cells of the lymphocyte/histiocytic or popcorn-cell type.
- In mixed-cellularity HD, the infiltrate is of classic RS cells and their mononuclear variants together with lymphocytes, plasma cells, eosinophils and histiocytes.
- As the name implies, nodes affected by nodular sclerosing HD show division of the node by bands of collagen. The RS cells present show artefactual retraction of their cytoplasm leading to the lacunar RS-cell variant. If the infiltrate is similar to that seen in mixed-cellularity, then the node is said to show type I disease. If abundant pleomorphic RS cells are seen however, it is classified as type II.
- In lymphocyte-depleted HD the infiltrate is composed of abundant plemorphic RS cells.

2 Ann Arbor Staging System
Stage I – Disease confined to one group of lymph nodes or extranodal site (IE).

Stage II – Disease confined to several nodal groups on the same side of the diaphragm with limited involvement of an adjacent extranodal site (IIE).

Stage III – Disease is present in lymph node groups on both sides of the diaphragm or with limited involvement of an adjacent extranodal site (IIIE) or with involvement of the spleen (IIIS).

Stage IV – Disseminated involvement of one or more extranodal tissue, such as the liner or bone marrow, with or without nodal involvement.

These groups are further subdivided on the absence (A) or presence (B) or symptoms which include: unexplained fever (above 38°C), night sweats and unexplained weight loss of greater than 10% of body weight in the preceding six months.

3 Prognosis
The best prognosis is seen with lymphocyte-predominant HD and nodular-sclerosis grade I, the worst with lymphocyte-depleted HD and nodular sclerosis grade II. The prognosis in mixed-cellularity HD is largely dependent on stage at time of diagnosis. Bad prognostic features within each subgroup include increasing age, increasing stage and the presence of B symptoms.

CASE 41

Mr Zak Wormold, a 72-year-old retired pest-control officer, is admitted to hospital as an emergency. He lives alone and has been has been found by a man who called to read the electricity meter. He is confused and is complaining of severe back pain. His daughter arrives and tells you that when she saw her father a week ago he was complaining that he was drinking a lot and could not stop going to the toilet to pass urine. Physical examination reveals pallor but nothing otherwise. The results of the initial investigations are as follows:

Investigation	Result
Hb	9 g/dl ($\downarrow$)
WBC	$6.8 \times 10^9/l$
Platelets	$150 \times 10^9/l$
Corrected Ca^{2+}	3.8 mmol/l ($\uparrow\uparrow$)
ESR	60 mm/hr ($\uparrow\uparrow$)
Creatinine	120 mmol/l ($\uparrow$)
Lumbar-spine X-ray	Multiple punched-out lytic lesions seen in ribs and vertebral bodies

A diagnosis of myeloma is confirmed by further investigations. In the subsequent months the patient's renal function gradually declines.

Questions

1 How is the diagnosis of myeloma confirmed?
2 What are the possible causes of a decline in renal function?
3 This patient's symptoms were caused by destruction of bone and hypercalcaemia. What is the other major cause of symptoms in myeloma?

YOUR ANSWERS

1 Diagnosis of myeloma confirmed

2 Renal function in myeloma

3 Other problems

CASE 41 ANSWERS   pp. 295, 296

1 Diagnosis of myeloma confirmed

Although the clinical features and X-ray findings in combination with a raised ESR and raised Ca^{2+} are highly suggestive of myeloma, the diagnosis must be confirmed by serum electrophoresis for the detection of a monoclonal immunoglobulin protein (paraprotein) and bone marrow biopsy to detect an increased number of monoclonal plasma cells. The infiltrate of abnormal antibody-producing plasma cells may be patchy or diffuse.

The paraprotein itself is most often of the IgG class (50%) and restricted to the Kappa light-chain variety (60%). Bence–Jones Proteins (composed of light chains only) may be found in the urine. Rarely, myeloma may be non-secretory i.e., producing no paraprotein.

2 Renal function in myeloma

There are many possible causes of renal failure in myeloma and several are readily reversible. They include:

- Dehydration.
- Hypercalcaemia.
- Hyperuricaemia.
- Urinary-tract infection.
- Damage to tubular epithelium by light-chain casts.
- Infiltration of kidney by plasma cells.
- Amyloid.

3 Other problems

One of the major problems in myeloma is the paraprotein. In the presence of high levels of this protein the production of normal gammaglobulin is reduced, leading to recurrent bacterial infections. The abnormal protein can also give rise to a hyperviscosity syndrome, especially with the IgM and IgG3 types which may aggregate. The hyperviscosity syndrome presents clinically with fatigue, headaches, focal neurological deficits and fits. Patients may also develop retinal haemorrhages and papilloedema. A bleeding tendency or hypercoagulable state may occur as a result of a paraprotein.

CASE 42

Luke Wainscott is a two-year-old boy who has been brought to see you because his mother is worried about his health. Marie Wainscott, his mother, is a single parent, living in a refuge for battered wives. Over the previous four days, Luke, who was previously well, has had a temperature, been off his food, and today has come out in red spots with bleeding gums. Examination reveals a petechial skin rash, generalized lymphadenopathy and mild splenomegaly. A diagnosis of acute leukaemia is made.

Questions

1 How might one disease process explain this complex of symptoms?
2 How is a specific diagnosis achieved?
3 How are acute leukaemias classified?

YOUR ANSWERS

1 Explanation of symptoms and signs

2 Diagnosis

3 Classification of acute leukaemias

CASE 42 ANSWERS pp. 292, 293

1 Explanation of symptoms and signs

In acute leukaemia, replacement of bone marrow by blast cells causes loss of red-cell production, leading to anaemia and the associated symptoms. Granulopoiesis (white-cell production) is impaired, leading to susceptibility to infections. Megakaryocytopoiesis (platelet production) is impaired, leading to a bleeding tendency.

2 Diagnosis

The peripheral blood will show an increased white-cell count in about half of the cases of acute leukaemia. The diagnosis is established by bone marrow aspirate or trephine biopsy which will show extensive replacement of normal haemopoietic tissue by abnormal blast cells.

3 Classification of acute leukaemia

Acute leukaemias are broadly divided into:

- Acute lymphoblastic leukamia (ALL) seen mostly in children.
- Acute non-lymphoblastic leukaemia (ANLL) seen most often in adults.

In ALL, the morphology (FAB type) of the leukaemic cells and the presence or absence of specific cell-surface antigens allows a prognosis to be given.

The ANLL's are divided into eight FAB types with varying degrees of granulocytic, erythroid or megakaryocytic differentiation of the blast cells.

7

ENDOCRINE SYSTEM

CASE 43

Mr Robert Trustone is a 42-year-old salesman. He works for a company selling electrical equipment to measure sulphur emissions from incinerator chimneys and spends much of his time driving around the country. He comes to see his doctor because he has been getting increasingly severe headaches for about a month. He has also been feeling very tired. The day before, he backed his car into a wall which he hadn't noticed and he feels that there is something wrong with his vision. He says that he has never suffered from migraine.

On examination he is found to have a visual defect: bitemporal hemianopia but no papilloedema is present. The rest of the examination is normal.

He is urgently admitted to the Neurosurgery Department where investigations revealed a large non-functioning pituitary adenoma for which he is treated by trans-sphenoidal hypophysectomy.

Questions

1 What investigations would be useful?
2 What is the cause of the visual defect?

YOUR ANSWERS

1 Investigations

2 Cause of visual failure

CASE 44

Mrs Georgina Hall is a 30-year-old housewife who is seen by her doctor because her sister had told her that she was looking a bit thin. She tells you that she has indeed lost weight in spite of a good appetite. When you question her you notice that she has exophthalmos. On examination, her thyroid gland is diffusely enlarged and her pulse is 100 with atrial fibrillation.

Questions

1 What is the likely diagnosis?
2 What single initial investigation would be most useful?
3 What is the most likely pathogenesis of her condition?

YOUR ANSWERS

1 Diagnosis

2 Useful test

3 Most likely pathogenesis

CASE 43 ANSWERS p. 299

1 Investigations

The investigations are listed below together with the appropriate results.

Investigation	Result
CT/MRI scans	Enlargement of sella turcica and erosion of posterior clinoid process. Pituitary-gland tumour showing suprasellar extension
Pituitary-function tests	No evidence of hyper- or hypopituitarism
Visual-field assessment	Bitemporal hemianopia is present

2 Cause of visual failure

The optic chiasm is a structure situated above the pituitary gland which transmits nerve fibres from the optic nerves of both eyes towards the optic tracts and eventually to the occipital visual cortex. A pituitary tumour which extends above the sella turcica is able to compress the optic chiasm producing bitemporal hemianopia.

CASE 44 ANSWERS p. 303

1 Diagnosis

The patient has the clinical features of hyperthyroidism. The presence of exophthalmos is a characteristic feature of Graves' disease. Other clinical features are pretibial myxoedema, acropachy (clubbing), splenomegaly and lymphadenopathy.

2 Useful test

Thyroid function tests would allow confirmation of hyperthyroidism thus allowing appropriate treatment of the patient.

Thyroid Function Test	Result
TSH	Low
Thyroxine (T4)	Raised

3 Most likely cause and pathogenesis

The most likely cause in a woman this age is Graves' disease, an autoimmune disorder where a stimulating IgG antibody called LATS (also called thyroid-stimulating immunoglobulin) is produced which binds to thyroid acinar cells, mimicking the effects of TSH, and resulting in excess thyroxine production. The normal hormonal feedback mechanism is bypassed. It is the commonest cause of hyperthyroidism, typically occurring in middle-aged females. It is often associated with other autoimmune disorders such as IDDM and pernicious anaemia.

CASE 45

Ms Jocelyn Peabody is a 25-year-old woman, recently set up in a small business refurbishing old rocking horses and other large pieces of nursery equipment. She has been sent to hospital for assessment because her family doctor is worried about a lump in her neck. The lump had become obvious as a vague discomfort when she was applying skin cream and had been increasing in size over the previous two months. She felt well otherwise. On examination, a hard 3cm nodule is felt in the left lobe of her thyroid gland together with adjacent cervical lymphadenopathy.

Investigations are performed and a papillary carcinoma of the thyroid gland is diagnosed and treated.

Questions

1 What is the differential diagnosis of a nodule in the thyroid?
2 What investigations would you have performed to assess the thyroid nodule?
3 What features in the history are suggestive of carcinoma?
4 What is her prognosis?

YOUR ANSWERS

1 Diagnosis

2 Investigations

3 Features suggesting carcinoma

4 Prognosis

CASE 46

Mr Daniel Dare is a 40-year-old airline pilot who, 15 years before, had initially trained as a fighter pilot. He is being seen because he has had several 'odd episodes' over a period of three weeks. He describes attacks, each one lasting approximately twenty minutes, where he develops severe headaches, thumping of his heart, sweating, nausea, tremor and feeling faint. His past medical history includes a parathyroid gland adenoma which was removed surgically 10 years previously.

On examination, the only positive finding is hypertension: BP= 180/100.

Questions

1 What is the likely diagnosis?
2 How would you confirm the diagnosis?
3 What is the significance of the patient's previous parathyroid adenoma?

YOUR ANSWERS

1 Likely diagnosis

2 Investigations

3 Significance of adenoma

CASE 45 ANSWERS pp. 304, 305

1 Diagnosis

Solitary nodules in the thyroid may be a disproportionately large nodule of a multinodular goitre, a thyroid adenoma, or a malignant thyroid tumour.

2 Investigations

A list of appropriate investigations with the results are given below:

Investigation	Result
Thyroid-function tests	Normal
Thyroglobulin	Raised
Radioactive-iodine scan	An inactive or 'cold' nodule
Ultrasound scan	The nodule is solid in consistency
FNA cytology	Malignant cells typical of papillary-cell carcinoma are present
Chest CT	No tracheal compression or retrosternal extension of tumour is seen

3 Features suggesting carcinoma

A short clinical history and an asymmetrically enlarged hard thyroid nodule with adjacent cervical lymphadenopathy are all suggestive of cancer.

Although not present in this patient, the presence of pressure symptoms, e.g. stridor and hoarseness should alert one to possible carcinoma.

4 Prognosis

A total thyroidectomy would be recommended because of the multifocal nature of papillary carcinoma of the thyroid. Subsequent metastatic disease can be monitored with serum thyroglobulin levels and whole body iodine uptake scans. It can be treated with high dose I^{131}. Thyroxine would be given post-operatively to replace loss of endogenous thyroxine and also to suppress any residual tumour growth by directly suppressing TSH release by the anterior pituitary via a negative feedback mechanism. Papillary-cell carcinoma has a good prognosis in young people with a 80% survival of five years.

CASE 46 ANSWERS pp. 311, 312, 315

1 Likely diagnosis

The clinical history is suggestive of a phaeochromocytoma which is a rare but treatable cause of hypertension. It is a tumour of the sympathetic nervous system, the majority of which occur in the adrenal gland. The chromaffin cells of the adrenal medulla secrete noradrenaline and adrenaline which accounts for the symptoms.

2 Investigations

- 24-hour urinary collection for catecholamines/VMA/meta-adrenalins.
- CT/MRI scan of abdomen to localize the lesion.

Thyroid-Function Test	Result
24-hour urinary collection	Raised levels of NA, VMA and HMMA
MRI Scan	Large left-side adrenal mass is present

3 Significance of adenoma

A phaeochromocytoma is a component of multiple endocrine neoplasia II or MEN II which occurs in association with parathyroid tumours and medullary cell carcinoma of thyroid gland. The patient has had a previous parathyroid adenoma so a medullary cell carcinoma of the thyroid needs to be excluded. The patient did not have a thyroid carcinoma as evidenced by clinical examination and a normal serum calcitonin. He should have his calcitonin level assessed periodically.

8

URINARY SYSTEM

CASE 47

Kate Rowntree is a 13-year-old girl who is brought by her parents because she had become lethargic and her face appeared swollen, particularly around her eyes. On enquiry, she had recently recovered from a flu-like illness. As part of routine examination her urine is tested with a dip-stick and is found that to contain both protein and blood. She is also noted to have a mildly raised blood pressure.

The patient is referred to hospital where she is found to have raised urea and creatinine together with a reduced urine output. Renal biopsy is performed.

The histology report reveals hypercellularity of glomeruli with neutrophils in capilary lumina. Granular deposition of IgG, C1q and C3 are seen in the glomerular basement membrane and mesangium. Electron microscopy confirms the presence of electron dense deposits in the basement membrane, predominantly in a subepithelial location.

Questions

1 What clinical syndrome does she have?
2 What investigations do pathologists perform on renal biopsy tissue and why?
3 What is the most likely diagnosis in this case?
4 What is her prognosis?

CASE 47 ANSWERS   pp. 319, 325, 326, 327

1 Clinical syndrome

She has the nephritic syndrome – oliguria, haematuria, uraemia and raised blood pressure.

2 Investigation of the renal biopsy

- Routine histology to look at changes in glomeruli, interstitium and tubules.
- Immunofluorescence or immunohistochemistry are performed to look for deposits of different types of immunoglobulin and complement components, either within the glomerular-capillary basement membrane or the mesangium. Special histochemical staining allows more detailed analysis of which components of the glomerulus have been affected by the disease process. This is done to define different types of immune-mediated glomerular damage.
- Electron microscopy can confirm the presence of immune deposits and identifies the exact site of complex deposition. If no complexes are present, other abnormalities of the basement membrane or adjacent cells may be evident.

3 Diagnosis

Acute diffuse proliferative glomerulonephritis (acute post-infective glomerulonephritis).

4 Prognosis

Providing the patient can be supported through the acute phase of the illness, complete resolution is the usual outcome. However, a small proportion of patients may develop diffuse crescentic glomerulonephritis with rapidly progressive decline in renal function, and a similar small percentage may apparently recover fully, except for persistent proteinuria, and develop chronic renal failure may years later.

CASE 48

Matthew Swan is a four-year-old boy who is referred to hospital by his family doctor. He has presented with generalized oedema and is found to have heavy proteinuria (4.1 g/l) and hypoalbuminaemia. A renal biopsy shows no abnormality on routine light microscopy.

Questions

1 What syndrome has this child presented with?
2 What is the probable diagnosis?
3 What further investigation may be helpful and what would confirm your diagnosis?
4 Is this condition treatable, if so how and what is the prognosis?

YOUR ANSWERS

1 Syndrome

2 Diagnosis

3 Confirming diagnosis

4 Treatment and prognosis

CASE 49

Mr Cuthbert Digby is a 57-year-old draughtsman who presents to his family practitioner complaining of a dragging sensation in his left loin. On questioning, he admits to having had intermittent painless haematuria for three weeks. Following referral to a urological surgeon, investigation reveals a large mass replacing the left kidney. He undergoes a left nephrectomy from which he makes a good recovery.

Questions

1 What is the most likely diagnosis?
2 What is the most common histological pattern of this lesion and what causes this appearance?
3 What factors in the histopathologists report would have a particular bearing on the prognosis for this patient?
4 What is the natural history for these lesions if untreated?

YOUR ANSWERS

1 Diagnosis

2 Common histological pattern

3 Prognosis features

4 Natural history

CASE 48 ANSWERS pp. 319, 332, 336

1 Syndrome

Nephrotic syndrome (proteinuria, oedema, hypoalbuminaemia)

2 Diagnosis

In this age group, minimal change glomerulonephritis is by far the most likely diagnosis. Less common would be focal glomerulosclerosis, membranoproliferative glomerulonephritis, and proliferative glomerulonephritis.

3 Confirming diagnosis

Light microscopy is usually normal, but electron microscopy frequently shows morphological abnormalities of the epithelial cells. Either fusion of the foot processes occurs (podocytes) or withdrawal of the foot processes so that the epithelial cell body is sitting directly on the glomerular basement membrane.

4 Treatment and prognosis

The condition normally responds over a period of weeks to treatment with corticosteroids; the long term outlook is excellent.

CASE 49 ANSWERS pp. 341, 342

1 Diagnosis

The most likely diagnosis is renal carcinoma.

2 Common histological pattern

Carcinomas of the kidney are adenocarcinomas. The most common histological pattern is of a clear-cell pattern which is due to accumulation of lipid and glycogen within the cytoplasm of neoplastic cells.

3 Prognostic features

If carcinoma is present within blood vessels (particularly the renal veins) at the hilum, then there is a greater likelihood that metastatic spread will ensue. If tumour is confined within the renal capsule there is a 70% 10-year survival.

4 Natural history

If untreated, tumour extends locally by invasion through the renal capsule to involve local structures. Blood-borne metastasis is common, particularly to bone, lung and brain. Metastatic renal carcinoma is resistant to treatment.

CASE 50

Mr Joe Spearman has been referred to see you because an insurance medical has revealed that he has very high blood pressure. He is 45 years old and has just achieved a business breakthrough marketing replacement hard drives for personal computers. His blood pressure is confirmed to be high at 140/100. Going into his family history, it transpires that his father had died of a stroke at about the same age and he remembers something vague about him having had 'large kidneys'.

Questions

1 What disease does this patient have?
2 What is its mode of inheritance?
3 How would you confirm the diagnosis?
4 Give two possible causes of his fathers 'stroke'.
5 What other features are associated with the condition?

YOUR ANSWERS

1 Diagnosis

2 Inheritance

3 Confirming diagnosis

4 Causes of stroke in father

5 Other associated features

CASE 51

Mr Charles Ramsbottom was attending his retirement partly after 40 years of unbroken service as a tyre presser at the ATKA rubber factory in Burnley when he had fallen into conversation with an old friend. He remarked that he had been a little taken aback because his water had turned red during the last month. He said he was glad to be retiring as he was beginning to feel rather 'washed out'. His friend advised him to go and see his doctor as it sounded serious.

Questions

1 Why is Charles feeling 'washed out'?
2 What would his peripheral blood film show?
3 What is the probable diagnosis?
4 How should he be investigated?
5 Why has he developed this disease?

YOUR ANSWERS

1 Reason for feeling tired

2 Blood film

3 Diagnosis

4 Investigation

5 Aetiology

CASE 50 ANSWERS pp. 348, 349

1 Diagnosis

Secondary hypertension due to adult polycystic disease of the kidney.

2 Inheritance

Adult polycystic disease of the kidney is inherited as an autosomal dominant trait. There are two main types, with the genes located on chromosome 16 and chromosome 2.

3 Confirming diagnosis

The kidneys in this condition are often extremely large by adulthood and so would be easily seen on abdominal ultrasound. They also should be palpable on routine physical examination.

4 Causes of stroke in his father

Adult polycystic disease of the kidney is associated with the development of berry aneurysms. His father may have developed one of these with subsequent rupture predisposed by his hypertension. Patients who are hypertensive are at increased risk of haemorrhagic strokes due to rupture of Charcot–Bouchard microaneurysms which develops secondary to hypertension.

5 Other associated features

As well as saccular aneurysms, there may be aortic dilatation causing aortic incompeteance and mitral valve prolapse. Cysts may be present in liver, pancreas and spleen. Colonic diverticular disease is common.

CASE 51 ANSWERS pp. 346, 347

1 Reason for feeling tired

He is probably anaemic from blood loss due to chronic haematuria.

2 Blood film

Hypochromic microcytic red cells. A raised reticulocyte count may be seen as his bone marrow attempts to deal with the red-cell loss.

3 Diagnosis

The most likely diagnosis is transitional-cell carcinoma arising in the urothelium. The commonest site would be the bladder.

4 Investigation

The first investigation should be a mid-stream urine specimen to exclude an infective cause, and three early morning urine samples. Cystoscopy allows complete visualization of the bladder mucosa and, in addition, abnormal areas should be biopsied for histological examination. If the lesions present are superficial, resection via the cystoscope may be adequate treatment. Repeat cystoscopy, with or without cystological analysis of urine, is normal in the following of such patients. If no tumour is seen in the bladder, investigation of the renal pelvis and ureters would be required.

5 Aetiology

Transitional-cell carcinoma is caused by the excretion in urine of carcinogens that are derived from environmental exposure. Smoking, working with aniline dyes, and working in the rubber industry are important predisposing causes. In this case, the fact that this person has been a lifelong worker at a tyre plant is important. He would be entitled to compensation having developed an occupational-related disease. In many instances, industries have implemented screening of workers by urinary cytology.

CASE 52

Ms Marjorie von Damelung is a 62-year-old, gifted viola teacher. She has a long history of urinary tract infections, and has been referred by her family doctor for a urological opinion because of a gradually worsening ache in her right loin over a period of six months. On plain abdominal X-ray, there is an obvious area of opacity which appears to be filling a distended pelvicalyceal system. An intravenous urogram shows normal function in her left kidney, but virtually no passage of contrast through her right kidney.

Questions

1 What name is given to the structure filling her right pelvicalyceal system?
2 What is its composition?
3 With what sort of organisms is it associated?
4 What are the different types of renal calculi?

Your answers

1 Structure in the renal pelvis

2 Composition

3 Associated organisms

4 Types of renal calculi

CASE 52 ANSWERS p. 345

1 Structure in the renal pelvis
A staghorn calculus or triple-phosphate stone.

2 Composition
Magnesium, ammonium, and calcium phosphates.

3 Associated organisms
Urea-splitting organisms which maintain an alkaline urine.

4 Types of renal calculi
- Calcium oxalate or phosphate stones – the most common type (80%).
- Magnesium, ammonium, and calcium phosphates – as in this case (15%).
- Uric acid stones (5%).
- Cystine stones (<1%).

9

MALE GENITAL SYSTEM

CASE 53

Timothy Twist is a 14-year-old adolescent male, who is a keen soccer player. He is brought to the emergency department by his parents having woken in the night with severe pain in his scrotum. On examination he is systemically well but in obvious distress. The right side of the scrotum appears swollen, congested and remarkably tender to palpation. He underwent an exploratory operation.

Questions

1 What is the most likely diagnosis?
2 What other diagnoses would you consider?
3 What would the testis look like and how might this influence treatment?

CASE 54

Roger 'Bull' Crackman is a 24-year-old army corporal in a special operations unit. He reports to his medical officer that he has noticed a swelling in his scrotum. Initially, this had come to light while he was taking a shower after a four-day field endurance exercise and he had put it down to chaffing from his kit. However, the swelling had not gone down and had enlarged over the past two months. On examination, he has a non-tender left-sided hydrocele from which bloodstained fluid is aspirated. The medical officer thinks that the underlying testis may be slightly enlarged, but is uncertain and refers the patient for specialist opinion.

Questions

1 What is the most likely diagnosis?
2 What further investigations would be appropriate?

YOUR ANSWERS

1 Likely diagnosis

2 Other diagnoses

3 Appearance of testis

YOUR ANSWERS

1 Diagnosis

2 Investigations

CASE 53 ANSWERS pp. 350, 351

1 Likely diagnosis
Torsion of the testis.

2 Other diagnoses
- Torsion of a testicular appendage, e.g. hydatid of morgagni.
- An acute epididymo-orchitis.
- Involvement of an inguinal hernia, which communicates with the tunica vaginalis by a loop of small bowel.

3 Appearance of testis
In early torsion, the testis would appear swollen and suffused with blood. Early intervention at this stage with untwisting of the testicular pedicle may save the testis. Surgical intervention should also stabilize the testis to prevent recurrence. If neglected, torsion causes venous infarction leading to a swollen, almost black-coloured testis. If intervention is too late, and venous infarction has occurred, then orchidectomy is performed.

CASE 54 ANSWERS pp. 351, 357

1 Diagnosis
Acquired hydroceles are uncommon, and if they contain blood-stained fluid a malignant testicular neoplasm should be high on the list of differential diagnoses. At this age, with this presentation, the most likely diagnosis is a malignant teratoma of the testis.

2 Investigations
If the testis is not significantly enlarged, testicular ultrasound may identify a small tumour and indicate whether it is solid or cystic. Serum tumour cell markers (AFP – alpha fetoprotein and β-HCG – β-unit of human chorionic gonadotrophin) should be measured. If tumour is diagnosed, chest X-ray may show pulmonary metastases, especially with teratomas. Body imaging (CT or MRI) to identify stage and extent of tumour spread is now the ideal mode of investigation. Testicular tumours spread commonly to para-aortic and iliac lymph nodes, especially seminomas.

CASE 55

Mr Peter Churchill is a 74-year-old retired fruit-farm labourer. He says that he has been feeling unusually tired and has lost his appetite. Initial blood tests show that he is anaemic, with an Hb of 9.8 g/dl and has renal failure with a blood urea of 26 mmol/l and a creatinine of 280 mmol/l. On further enquiry, you find out that he has had a poor urinary stream, with some frequency, nocturia and a post-micturitional dribble. Rectal examination (PR) reveals a rubbery, firm, smooth enlargement of the prostate gland. Further investigations include an intravenous urogram (IVU) which showed both kidneys to be functioning but also showed bilateral hydronephrosis with hydroureter.

Questions

1 What is the most likely diagnosis?
2 What further tests may be helpful?
3 What abnormality is seen in the bladder?

YOUR ANSWERS

1 Diagnosis

2 Investigations

3 Changes in the bladder

CASE 56

Mr. Terence Westwood is a 50-year-old tree surgeon. He has come to seek medical attention complaining of inability to retract his foreskin fully. On examination, his foreskin shows thickening and scarring, and the glans, which is red and inflamed, shows pale atrophic patches.

Questions

1 What condition is the patient suffering from?
2 What problems have occurred secondary to this condition?

YOUR ANSWERS

1 Diagnosis

2 Complications

CASE 55 ANSWERS

pp. 344, 358, 359

1 Diagnosis

This person has renal failure caused by hydronephrosis as a result of obstruction of the prostatic urethra by an enlarged prostate gland. The smooth, rubbery gland makes it most likely that he has benign nodular prostatic hyperplasia. It is also possible that he has a carcinoma of the prostate.

2 Investigations

The serum-acid phosphatase and prostatic-specific antigen may be raised in prostatic carcinoma. Diagnostic assessment may be made by a per-rectum needle biopsy of the prostate.

3 Changes in the bladder

Obstruction of the bladder leads to thickening of the muscle and exaggeration of the trabecular pattern. Bladder diverticulae may develop.

CASE 56 ANSWERS

p. 360

1 Diagnosis

Balanitis xerotica obliterans – a condition in which there is scarring of the dermis causing phimosis. This is a primary inflammatory disorder of the skin which is also seen in the vulval region of women when it is known as lichen sclerosus.

2 Complications

The scarring has caused tightening of the foreskin which makes retraction difficult. This is known as phimosis and predisposes to poor hygiene giving rise to balanitis, and inflammation of the glans which is probably bacterial in origin.

10

GYNAECOLOGICAL AND OBSTETRIC PATHOLOGY

CASE 57

Mrs Jane Jenkins, a 32-year-old schoolmistress, presents to her gynaecologist with a four-year history of infertility. Her husband has been investigated and has a normal sperm count and normal sperm motility. On further questioning, she gives a history of lower abdominal pain premenstrually, as well as dysmenorrhoea, particularly in her sacral region, and also dyspareunia. On examination, she appears to be mildly tender in the region of the right ovary and small nodules (approximately 1 cm in diameter) are palpaple posterior to the uterus on vaginal examination. No other abnormality is found. Investigations show a normal haemoglobin, platelet and white cell count.

Laparoscopy is performed. The right ovary is enlarged and is fixed by adhesions to the Fallopian tube and broad ligament, with ill-defined dark-brown cystic areas. The posterior aspect of the uterus and the pouch of Douglas show similar cystic dark brown lesions up to 5 mm in their maximum extent.

The right ovary and Fallopian tube are excised and sent for histology. They show scattered cystic areas 3–5 cm in maximum dimension, containing thick brown fluid. Within the fibrous walls surrounding the cysts, endometrial glands and stroma are seen. Abundant macrophages containing haemosiderin pigment are present.

The appearances are those of pelvic and ovarian endometriosis.

Questions

1 What is the colloquial name often given to the ovarian cysts caused by endometriosis and why ?.
2 What are possible theories with regard to the pathogenesis of endometriosis?
3 What therapies may be used to treat the disease?

YOUR ANSWERS

1 Name given to cysts in endometriosis

2 Theories of pathogenesis of endometriosis

3 Treatment

CASE 57 ANSWERS
p. 371

1 Name given to cysts in endometriosis

The ovarian cysts of endometriosis are often called 'chocolate cysts' because of the colour and the consistency of the semi-viscous brown contents.

2 Theories of pathogenesis of endometriosis

The reason for the development of endometriosis is uncertain, but several theories have been proposed. These include:

- Retrograde menstruation (regurgitation or implantation theory). In normal women, fragments of endometrium may pass along the Fallopian tubes during menstruation and it has been suggested that this material may implant in women with endometriosis.
- Metaplasia of the peritoneal lining may produce foci of endometrial glands and stroma from the mesothelium normally lining the peritoneal cavity. This may also form tubal-type epithelium producing the related condition called endosalpingiosis.
- Metastatic spread of endometrium along lymphatics or blood vessels.

None of these theories explains all of the manifestations of endometriosis, nor what initiates the process in some women but not in others.

3 Treatment

The primary treatment is the suppression of the endometrial tissue by endocrine agents. Inducing a hypo-oestrogenic state with analogues of GnRH is often effective. Both the normal and the ectopic tissues respond to hormones, and the endometriotic focus undergoes the same cyclical changes as that within the uterus, causing the pain and the dark-brown colouration with haemosiderin pigment deposition due to bleeding. Surgery may be required, for example, to exclude other pathology when a mass lesion is produced or when symptoms do not respond, particularly in the older woman who has completed her family.

CASE 58

Mrs Josephine Noakes, a 67-year-old retired telephone operator, presents to her doctor with a five-month history of irregular postmenopausal bleeding. She has not been taking hormone replacement treatment. On examination, she appears pale. Vaginal examination shows no obvious local source for the bleeding. Full blood count shows a haemoglobin of 9.5 g/dl, with a normal white cell and platelet count.

Mrs Noakes undergoes dilatation and curettage which produces bulky uterine curettings. An enlarged right ovary can be felt under anaesthetic but is not biopsied. Histological examination shows severe cytological and architectural atypia of the endometrium and a diagnosis of endometrial adenocarcinoma is made.

She has a hysterectomy with a cuff of vagina excised, and bilateral salpingo-oophorectomy. The operative specimen is sent for pathological examination. The uterine cavity is filled with focally necrotic, pale, friable tumour measuring approximately 7 cm in maximum dimension. This extends into the myometrium, up to, but not through, the serosal surface. The cervix is not infiltrated by carcinoma/tumour which does not extend into the Fallopian tubes. The right ovary is enlarged with a well-defined yellow tumour 4 cm in diameter with a firm cut surface. Histological examination confirms that the uterine tumour is a moderately differentiated (grade 2) endometrial adenocarcinoma of endometrioid type. The right ovarian tumour is a benign thecoma.

Questions

1 What is the association between the endometrial carcinoma and the ovarian thecoma?
2 How do endometrial carcinomas spread?
3 How are endometrial carcinomas staged and what is the prognosis, based on stage, for Mrs Noakes?

YOUR ANSWERS

1 Association between thecoma and endometrial carcinoma

2 Spread of endometrial carcinoma

3 Stage and prognosis

CASE 59

Ms Racquel Purvis, a 23-year-old "beautician" working at a local massage parlour and sauna, presents to her family doctor because she has developed a foul-smelling vaginal discharge. She complains of some associated vulval and vaginal itching and soreness. She is otherwise well. On examination, the vaginal and cervical mucosa are reddened, and a frothy, white, fishy-smelling discharge is noted. A high vaginal swab is taken.

Microscopic examination showed motile flagellated protozoa approximately 30 µm in maximum dimension. The appearances are those of infection with *Trichomonas vaginalis*.

Questions

1 What other organisms may cause vulval and vaginal infections?
2 How is *Trichomonas* usually transmitted?
3 What is the treatment?

YOUR ANSWERS

1 Other organisms causing vulvo–vaginal infection

2 Transmission

3 Treatment

CASE 58 ANSWERS   pp. 373, 380

1 Association between thecoma and endometrial carcinoma

The ovarian thecoma is a benign sex-cord stromal tumour which secretes oestrogens. Endometrial carcinoma (and endometrial hyperplasia) are linked to prolonged oestrogenic stimulation of the endometrium in post-menopausal women, and as many as 20% of post-menopausal women with ovarian thecomas develop endometrial carcinoma.

2 Spread of endometrial carcinoma

Carcinoma of the body of the uterus spreads locally into the myometrium and the depth of invasion has a close correlation with prognosis. Spread along the Fallopian tube may lead to ovarian metastases. Lymphatic spread occurs when the myometrium is deeply infiltrated, with consequent internal iliac and para-aortic lymph node metastases. Venous spread is less common but is thought to give rise to low vaginal metastases which are seen occasionally.

3 Stage and prognosis

Stage I carcinomas are confined to the body of the uterus, and patients have a 75% five-year survival. Mrs Noakes' tumour falls within this group. Stage II carcinomas of the endometrium have, in addition, infiltrated into the cervix and the five-year survival falls to 52%. Stage III carcinomas involve the side walls of the pelvis and have a 30% five-year survival and stage IV carcinomas have spread outside the pelvis or involve the rectum or the bladder and have a very poor (approximately 10%) five-year survival.

CASE 59 ANSWERS   p. 363

1 Other organisms causing vulvo–vaginal infection

Other common causes of lower, female, genital-tract infections include *Candida albicans, Gardnerella vaginalis, Herpes simplex, Gonococcus, Mycoplasma* and Human Papilloma Virus. *Staphylococci* may less commonly give rise to toxic-shock syndrome when proliferation, often in a retained tampon, occurs. Syphilitic infections are increasingly uncommon.

2 Transmission

Trichomonas vaginalis is usually sexually transmitted.

3 Treatment

Metronidazole is the present treatment of choice for urogenital trichomonas infections.

CASE 60

Mrs Anita Butcher, a 35-year-old sales assistant at a discount frozen-food warehouse, attends her doctor for a routine cervical smear. She is asymptomatic and well, but has not visited her doctor for the previous five years and has not had a smear in that time.

The cervical cytological report shows severe dyskaryosis.

She is recalled and has colposcopy performed which demonstrates the abnormal area of the cervical squamous epithelium which is biopsied. The changes seen colposcopically extend up the endocervical canal, and the upper margin of the abnormality can not be seen.

Histology shows that this is indeed an area of CIN (cervical intraepithelial neoplasia) grade 3, at the transformation zone, with atypical cells extending through the full thickness of the epithelium and showing no maturation towards the surface. Mitotic figures, including abnormal forms, are present through all layers. There is no evidence of invasion in the biopsy.

Mrs Butcher then has a cone biopsy performed. This confirms that CIN 3 is present at the transformation zone. There is no evidence of invasive squamous-cell carcinoma, no glandular atypia and the severe atypia is completely excised at both ecto- and endocervical margins.

Questions

1 If Mrs Butcher had not had the disease identified by screen ing what would have been her risk of developing invasive cervical carcinoma?
2 What are the risk factors for developing cervical carcinoma?

YOUR ANSWERS

1 Risk of developing invasive cervical carcinoma if CIN 3 present

2 Risk factors for cervical carcinoma

CASE 61

Mrs Jenny Mills, a 41-year-old woman who runs her own home-made vegetable pie business, presents to her doctor complaining of heavy periods. She is otherwise well, and her menstrual cycle is regular. She has one child and does not want more. On examination she is pale and has a bulky irregularly shaped uterus. Her ovaries are both palpable and bulky.

Her haemoglobin is 9.9 g/dl, her white cell and platelet counts are normal.

She is admitted to hospital for a routine hysterectomy which reveals a grossly enlarged irregular uterus. Macroscropic examination shows multiple, well-defined, rubbery, pale tumours of the myometrium, with a whorled cut surface. The largest measures 12 cm in maximum dimension. Histological examination confirms that these are leiomyomas (fibroids).

Questions

1 What are the possible presentations and complications of leiomyomas?
2 How is a leiomyoma distinguished from a leiomyosarcoma?

YOUR ANSWERS

1 Presentation of leiomyomas

2 Diagnosis from leiomyosarcoma

CASE 60 ANSWERS
pp. 367, 368

1 Risk of developing invasive cervical cancer if CIN 3 present

CIN is a precursor of carcinoma of the cervix, but not all cases would progress to invasive disease. The risk of this happening, however, appears to be higher with CIN 3 than lesser grades of atypia. It has been predicted that 20% of patients with CIN 3 would progress to develop invasive carcinoma within 10 years (35–40% within 20 years). Conversely 50% of women with CIN 1 have spontaneous regression of the disease, but 20% will progress through CIN 2 to CIN 3 over a period of 10 years. It is thus important to treat and follow up all women with cervical atypia.

2 Risk factors for cervical carcinoma

Risk factors for developing squamous-cell carcinoma of the cervix include:

- Human papilloma virus infection – currently an area of great interest, HPV 16, 18 and 33 have been found in more than 60% of cases of cervical carcinoma, suggesting a link and possibly a causative effect. It is believed that proteins produced by HPV inactivate tumour-suppressor genes, thus facilitating tumour development or progression.
- Sexual intercourse – a very low incidence is seen in virgins.
- Age at first intercourse – there is a higher incidence in those who have sex before the age of 17 and in those who marry early.
- Socioeconomic status – a higher incidence is seen in lower social groups, but this may be related to life style and sexual habits.
- Smoking.
- HIV infection.

CASE 61 ANSWERS
pp. 374, 375

1 Presentation of leiomyomas

Leiomyomas usually present with abnormal, often heavy, menstrual bleeding and consequent anaemia. They can cause subfertility or, during pregnancy, may result in spontaneous abortion or premature or obstructed labour. During pregnancy, they may also undergo necrobiosis causing pain. Occasionally, if very large, they can have a compression effect, for example on the bladder causing urinary frequency. Pedunculated fibroids may undergo torsion and infarct. Malignant change is thought to be very rare in leiomyomas, and most malignant smooth muscle tumours arise *de novo*.

2 Diagnosis from leiomyosarcoma

A leiomyoma is recognized by a lack of cellular atypia and mitoses. Leiomyosarcomas have an increased cellularity, with nuclear hyperchromatism and mitoses; the latter feature is the most important. Occasionally, it may be difficult to determine the biological behaviour of a smooth-muscle tumour, and it must be placed into the group termed as having 'uncertain malignant potential'.

CASE 62

Miss Georgina Blenkinsop, a 29-year-old intensive-care nurse, presents as an emergency to hospital with acute abdominal pain. Her menstrual cycle has been regular and she has had a period nine days earlier. She is tender in the right iliac fossa and, on bimanual examination, a mass thought to be ovarian in origin can be palpated. Her full blood count is normal and a pregnancy test is negative.

She has a laparotomy and a haemorrhagic right ovarian mass is removed. In addition, her left ovary contains a smaller tumour and this was also resected. She makes an uneventful recovery. The removed ovarian tissue is sent for pathological examination.

Macroscopic examination reveals bilateral cystic ovarian tumours: the larger right tumour measuring 8 cm in maximum extent. This has a purple, haemorrhagic appearance and, on opening, is unilocular, containing greasy material, teeth and hair. Histology confirms that both are bilateral benign cystic teratomas (dermoid cysts) with mature bone, muscle, neural and respiratory and skin elements also seen.

Questions

1 How common are mature cystic teratomas of the ovary?
2 Why did Miss Blenkinsop present with abdominal pain?
3 What are the other complications of ovarian mature cystic-teratomas?
4 What are the other four types of germ-cell tumour and what is their behaviour?

YOUR ANSWERS

1 How common are cystic ovarian teratomas

2 Reason for acute abdominal pain

4 Complications of cystic ovarian teratomas

3 Germ-cell tumour classification

CASE 63

Mrs Venetia Snodgrass, a 29-year-old teacher of Italian, develops bleeding per vaginam in the ninth week of pregnancy. She has abdominal 'cramps' and, by the time she has reached hospital, has passed several large haemorrhagic tissue fragments. She continues to bleed PV. On examination, the cervical os is dilated. Mrs Snodgrass is given intravenous fluids, and a dilatation and curettage are performed. Scanty material only is recovered and sent for histology.

Histological examination confirms that features of products of conception are present, including decidua and trophoblastic tissue. There is no evidence of an infective agent histologically.

Questions

1 What proportion of fertilized ova fail to implant successfully?
2 What are the causes of first-trimester spontaneous abortions?

YOUR ANSWERS

1 What proportion of fertilized ova fail to implant successfully?

2 What are the causes of first-trimester spontaneous abortions?

CASE 62 ANSWERS pp. 353, 381

1 How common are cystic ovarian teratomas

These are the most common ovarian germ-cell tumours, and account for about 10% of all ovarian neoplasms; 10% are bilateral. They occur in the reproductive age group and most are asymptomatic or incidental findings.

2 Reason for acute abdominal pain

The haemorrhagic appearance of the right-sided tumour is that of an ovarian mass which has undergone torsion and is becoming infarcted due to venous drainage obstruction; this can lead to rupture. If a rupture is less acute, and the sebaceous contents of the cyst are released, a chemical peritonitis may ensue. In a small proportion of cases, secondary malignant change may develop – usually a squamous-cell carcinoma. Rarely, mature cystic teratomas develop along only one embryological line and form monophyletic teratomas. The most common of these is the struma ovarii composed of mature thyroid tissue which may cause hyperthyroidism.

3 Germ-cell tumour classification

Germ-cell tumours may either show no evidence of differentiation or develop along embryonic, or extra-embryonic lines as trophoblast or yolk sac.

- **Solid teratomas** are mostly immature (malignant immature teratoma) and behave in a malignant fashion, implanting on the peritoneum and metastasizing via lymphatics and blood vessels.
- **Dysgerminoma** is the equivalent of the seminoma of the testis, and is formed of cells resembling primitive germ cells. These are malignant but radiosensitive tumours, with a good survival rate.
- **Yolk-sac tumours** are rare, occur in girls and young women and are highly malignant, although the prognosis is improving with the introduction of more effective chemotherapeutic regimes. The patients can be followed up by assessing blood levels of alpha fetoprotein which the tumour secretes.
- **Ovarian choriocarcinoma** is a rare form of germ-cell neoplasia that responds poorly to the chemotherapy which acts successfully on uterine choriocarcinomas. It has a propensity for vascular spread. Human chorionic gonadotrophin is secreted and can be used as a tumour marker.

CASE 63 ANSWERS p. 382

1 Proportion of ova failing to implant

It has been estimated that over 40% of conceptions fail to implant into the uterus and convert into recognized pregnancies. Another 15% of recognized pregnancies then also terminate as spontaneous abortions.

2 Causes of spontaneous first trimester abortions

The majority of spontaneous first-trimester abortions are due to fetal abnormality, most associated with abnormal chromosome karyotypes. Structural fetal abnormalities, such as neural tube defects, may also be a cause. Transplacental infections such as *Brucella, Listeria, Rubella, Toxoplasma*, cytomegalovirus and herpes virus infection may also lead to spontaneous abortions early in pregnancy. In addition, maternal systemic lupus erythematosus (SLE) and antiphospholipid antibody syndrome may induce repeated spontaneous abortions in the first trimester, and this condition may be clinically undiagnosed.

CASE 64

Mrs Flossie Harbottle, a 67-year-old retired greengrocer, presents to her doctor with a one-month history of a lump in the right breast. On examination, this is firm, ill-defined with skin tethering, and is adherent to the underlying pectoralis muscle. It measures approximately 4 cm in maximum extent. Within the right axilla, enlarged lymph nodes are palpable.

Fine-needle aspiration cytology (FNAC) confirms that carcinoma cells are present. Mrs Harbottle undergoes simple mastectomy with low axillary clearance. The operative specimens are sent for pathological examination.

Histological examination reveals a grade 3 invasive mammary adenocarcinoma of ductal type. Four out of eight axillary lymph nodes contained metastatic carcinoma.

Questions

1 What is the incidence of breast cancer?
2 What are the benefits of FNAC and what are the features of malignancy in a cytology preparation?
3 How, and to where, does breast carcinoma spread?

YOUR ANSWERS

1 Incidence of breast cancer

2 What are benefits of FNAC and what is seen in malignancy

3 Spread of breast cancer

CASE 65

Mrs Honoria Franklin, a 60-year-old geologist, attends for breast screening. She is in good health. A spiculate lesion is noted on her mammogram and she is recalled for assessment. No mass is palpable clinically. The radiological appearances are considered suspicious of carcinoma, and she undergoes stereotactic fine-needle aspiration cytology which reveals carcinoma cells. The lesion is localized by a marker wire and she has a therapeutic excision and lymph-node sampling. The operative samples are sent to pathology for analysis.

Histology reveals a small (0.9 cm maximum extent) grade 1 tubular carcinoma of the breast. The five axillary lymph nodes are free of tumour.

Questions

1 What histological features are assessed to determine histological grade of a breast carcinoma?
2 Apart from grade, what other features·can be useful in predicting prognosis in a woman with breast carcinoma?
3 What is Mrs Franklin's prognosis?

YOUR ANSWERS

1 Features used in grading breast cancer

2 Other prognostic features

3 Prognosis in this case

CASE 64 ANSWERS
pp. 391, 395, 396

1 Incidence of breast cancer

Breast cancer is the most common malignancy in women, with 1 in 10 women in the United States developing breast cancer at some time in their life (1 in 12 in the UK). It is second only to lung cancer in estimated cancer deaths, and its incidence is on the increase. Breast carcinoma may occur at any age but is rare in the first three decades of life, increasing in incidence with age thereafter.

2 What are the benefits of FNAC? What is seen in malignancy?

Fine-needle aspiration cytology is used as part of a 'triple approach' to diagnose breast lesions. It is relatively painless, complication-free and has an extremely low false-positive rate. Cytological features of malignancy include pleomorphism and increased cell size and loss of cohesion of the cells. In addition, carcinoma cells may have clumped chromatin and multiple prominent nucleoli. The smears are often more cellular than specimens from benign lesions.

3 Spread of breast cancer

Breast carcinomas spread locally into the overlying skin, causing tethering, and into the underlying pectoralis muscles, causing fixation. In addition, lymphatic and blood vessels may be invaded. In this way, tumour-cell emboli reach the local lymph nodes in the axilla and also the internal mammary node. Blood stream spread to bones may cause pathological fractures, spinal-cord compression and anaemia; spread to other organs may be seen including lung, pleura, ovary and brain.

CASE 65 ANSWERS
p. 395

1 Features used in grading breast cancer

Histological grade is determined by assessing three components of a breast carcinoma:

- The extent of the tumour which is forming tubules.
- The degree of pleomorphism and the cell size of the tumour cells.
- The mitotic count.

Some authorities use a method of assessing nuclear grade, instead of histological grade, which is also well-correlated with prognosis.

2 Other prognostic features

As well as histological grade, the staging of the tumour is of significance in predicting prognosis in patients with breast cancer. An accurate assessment of the size of the carcinoma is also predictive of outcome. Other variables of statistical significance in predicting survival are the presence or absence of vascular invasion and the histological type of carcinoma. Hormone receptor status is also related to prognosis, tumours expressing oestrogen receptors having a better prognosis than those that do not.

3 Prognosis in this case

Mrs Franklin has an excellent prognosis. She has a small, grade 1 carcinoma of tubular type with no evidence of metastases in her axillary lymph nodes. Her life expectancy is equivalent to that of an age-matched control, i.e. the same as if she had not had carcinoma.

CASE 66

Mrs Linda Bannister is a 44-year-old woman who presents to her doctor with an ill-defined area of lumpiness and pain in the left upper outer quadrant of breast. This has been causing her trouble ever since she began a parachute jumping course about two months ago. She is otherwise well. On taking a full history, she reports that she had always had menstrual irregularities, has never taken the oral contraceptive pill and has also noted some axillary tenderness recently. In the past, she has had breast pain, particularly premenstrually. On examination, she has multiple lumps in both breasts, several of which appear to be cystic in nature.

Fine-needle aspiration cytology is performed and cyst fluid is drained. This reveals sheets of benign cells showing apocrine metaplasia. A diagnosis of fibrocystic change (FCC) is made.

Questions

1 How common is fibrocystic change and what is the aetiology?
2 What are the histological components of fibrocystic change? Which of these features is important with respect to increased risk of developing breast carcinoma and how high is this risk?
3 What is the likely cause of Mrs Bannister's axillary tenderness?

CASE 66 ANSWERS pp. 388, 389

1 How common is fibrocystic change

Although it is impossible to give a precise incidence of fibrocystic change, it has been reported that over 40% of grossly normal breast that is examined histologically at autopsy show features of FCC. Clinical symptoms are said to be reported in 10% of women, often in their thirties or forties; few cases are seen in older patients who are not on hormone replacement treatment. It is now considered to be an exaggerated physiological response to relative excess or predominance of cycling oestrogenic hormones rather than a true disease; an increased incidence is seen in women with ovarian dysfunction and in those who have never taken the oral contraceptive pill.

2 Histology of fibrocystic disease and features related to cancer risk

As well as macroscopic cysts, microcystic change is often present. Apocrine metaplasia, adenosis, fibrosis and epithelial hyperplasia are also seen. The epithelial proliferation is the component which confers an increased risk of subsequent carcinoma developing. Epithelial hyperplasia of usual type confers a 1.5–2 fold increase in the risk of developing carcinoma. If this shows atypia (atypical ductal hyperplasia) the risk increases to 4–5 times that of the general population.

3 Reason for axillary tenderness

Mrs Bannister's axillary tenderness is most likely due to a reactive lymphadenopathy as a result of an inflammatory response to a ruptured breast cyst. This may have occurred from the rigours of parachute jumping. This clinical situation causes obvious diagnostic difficulties and malignancy must always be positively excluded by further investigation in a patient with a breast mass and enlarged lymph nodes.

12

NERVOUS SYSTEM AND MUSCLE

CASE 67

Barry 'Rat' Denzil is taken to the emergency room from an ambulance accompanied by his friends, members of a motor cycle gang called 'The Spores'. He has come off his bike on a bend and hit a tree. On examination, he is unconscious, making no response to painful stimuli. He was wearing a helmet which has come off in the accident. He has a fractured right femur and poor movement of the right side of his chest, with a clinical haemothorax. There is a bruise with a superficial laceration over the right temporal area of his scalp. Blood is coming out of his right ear. His right pupil is dilated and does not respond to light. His left pupil is of normal size and contracts in response to light.

He is intubated and ventilated, the haemothorax is drained, and he is made haemodynamically stable. A CT scan shows a right-sided extradural haematoma associated with a fracture of the temporal bone of the skull vault. An emergency operation is performed, and the extradural haematoma is evacuated. He is given intravenous mannitol and dexamethasone after the operation. However, his condition does not improve and, following appropriate criteria, he is pronounced brain-stem dead five days later.

Questions

1 What is the reason for a dilated and unreactive right pupil?
2 What is the origin of the extradural haematoma?
3 Why does he not make a recovery despite prompt treatment of the haematoma?
4 What is the clinical significance of the bleeding from the ear?

YOUR ANSWERS

1 Reason for dilated unreactive pupil

2 Origin of extradural haematoma

3 Reason for failure of recovery

4 Significance of bleeding from ear

CASE 67 ANSWERS   pp. 398, 405, 406

1 Reason for dilated unreactive pupil

The space-occupying haematoma on the right side has caused transtentorial herniation of the parahippocampal gyrus over the free edge of the tentorium cerebelli. This causes stretching of the third cranial nerve on the same side, resulting first in a sluggishly responding pupil, and then a paralysed dilated pupillary response. With further progression, the midbrain is compressed, leading to secondary midbrain haemorrhages.

2 Origin of extradural haematoma

The fracture of the skull has torn the middle meningeal artery, causing acute extradural haematoma.

3 Reason for failure of recovery

Brain pathology from head injury can be divided into two groups: primary and secondary. Secondary damage occurs after the inital impact and is caused by hypoxia, hypotension, and brain swelling. This patient has multiple trauma with unconsciousness, a haemothorax and a major leg fracture. It is therefore likely that he has sustained severe secondary brain damage.

4 Significance of bleeding from the ear

After head injury, bleeding from the ear strongly suggests a fracture of the base of the skull, usually involving the middle cranial fossa.

CASE 68

Mr Bertram Prempt is brought to hospital as an emergency, having collapsed at the bank where he is a financial advisor. He is unconscious and it is evident that he has a dense, left-sided hemiplegia. His wife attends and reveals that her husband, who is aged 63, has been on medication for high blood pressure for the past 10 years although he does not always take his tablets. His blood pressure is 150/100. ECG shows left ventricular hypertrophy. His full blood count is normal, as are measurements of serum urea and electrolytes. A CT scan shows a large haematoma, 3 cm in diameter, in the region of the right internal capsule/basal ganglia region.

Questions

1 What is the pathogenesis of this intracerebral haematoma?
2 What are the other common sites for hypertensive related haemorrhage in the brain?
3 What are other, less common, causes of intracerebral bleeding?

YOUR ANSWERS

1 Pathogenesis of haematoma?

2 Other common sites for hypertensive bleed in brain

3 Less common causes of intracerebral bleeding

CASE 69

Brian Crass is brought by his parents to the hospital emergency room. He is four years of age, and early in the afternoon had complained of being unwell and so was put to bed by his mother. Two hours later, when she had gone to check on how he was, his mother had found him virtually unrousable. On examination he is febrile and barely rousable, although is making responses to painful stimuli. He has marked neck stiffness. There are no focal neurological signs. Blood cultures are taken and high-dose dexamethasone is given just before high-dose intravenous antibiotics. A CT scan shows no mass lesion in the brain.

A lumbar puncture is performed. CSF is turbid and is sent for analysis. There are very large numbers of neutrophils. CSF sugar is low. Gram stain shows many Gram-negative cocco-bacilli with filamentous forms seen. A diagnosis of acute purulent meningitis is made and treatment started with appropriate antibiotics.

Questions

1 What organsisms commonly cause meningitis at this age?
2 What are the possible outcomes and complications following acute meningitis?

YOUR ANSWERS

1 Cause of meningitis at this age

2 Possible outcomes

CASE 68 ANSWERS p. 404

1 Pathogenesis of haematoma
The commonest cause of cerebral haemorrhage is hypertensive vascular damage. Prolonged hypertension results in arteriosclerosis and development of small micro-aneurysms, termed 'Charcot–Bouchard aneurysms', which predispose to vessel rupture, resulting in a haematoma.

2 Other common sites for hypertensive bleed in brain
The common sites for hypertensive intracerebral haematoma are the sites supplies by fine perforating vessels – basal ganglia, internal capsule, thalamus, cerebellum and pons.

3 Less common causes of intracerebral bleeding
In patients over the age of 70, 10% of cerebral haemorrhages are caused by the presence of cerebral artery amyloid composed of βA4 protein (amyloid angiopathy). This causes haematomas seen in the periphery of cerebral hemispheres (lobar haemorrhages).

Less common causes of a cerebral haematoma are bleeding into a tumour, rupture of vascular malformations, cerebral vasculitis, bleeding associated with disordered coagulation, and bleeding occurring in association with leukaemias.

CASE 69 ANSWERS p. 408

1 Causes of meningitis at this age
The main causes of acute purulent meningitis differ in different age groups:
- Neonates – *Escherichia coli, Streptococci, Listeria, monocytogenes.*
- Children – *Haemophilus influenzae, Neisseria meningitidis.*
- Adults – *Neisseria meningitidis, Streptococcus pneumoniae* type 3.
- Elderly – *Streptococcus pneumoniae* type 3, *Listeria monocytogenes.*

In this case, the age and Gram-negative coccobacilli suggest *Haemophilus influenzae* infection. The incidence of *Haemophilus* meningitis in children has fallen in areas with high uptake of Hib vaccination.

2 Possible outcomes
Acute bacterial meningitis is a severe life-threatening illness. Thrombosis of small cerebral vessels leads to diffuse cerebral ischaemic damage and death. If treated early, before vascular damage occurs, there may be resolution of disease but complications caused by organisation of the inflammatory exudate may lead to obstruction of the CSF drainage pathways and development of hydrocephalus. Cerebral abscess may also develop.

CASE 70

Mrs Elizabeth Handel, a 36-year-old farmers wife, is sent for a neurological opinion and investigation by her family doctor. She has developed weakness and incoordination of her right leg which is associated with some numbness. One year earlier, she had an episode of blurred vision associated with pain behind her right eye. Her doctor suspects that she might have multiple sclerosis.

On examination, she has loss of proprioception in her right leg associated with brisk reflexes and ankle clonus. She has reduced appreciation of light touch and pain in both legs. No other focal signs are seen.

Full blood count and ESR are normal. Seum B_{12} is normal. CSF shows a mild increase in lymphoid cells and a moderately elevated protein level. Electrophoresis of CSF shows oligoclonal immunoglobulin bands. Visual evoked potenials show delay of the positive wave in the right eye by 25 milliseconds, compared to the left which is normal. MRI scanning shows abnormal areas of signal in white matter at the angles of the lateral ventricles, in the cerebellar peduncles, and in the lower thoracic spinal cord.

A diagnosis of multiple sclerosis is made.

Questions

1 What is the pathogenesis of multiple sclerosis?
2 What is the name of the lesions and what do they look like?
3 What was the reason for the blurred vision and pain behind the eye?

YOUR ANSWERS

1 Pathogenesis of multiple sclerosis

2 Name and appearance of the lesions

3 Reason for blurred vision and eye pain

CASE 70 ANSWERS   pp. 413, 414

1 Pathogenesis of multiple sclerosis

Multiple sclerosis has a peak incidence between the ages of 20 and 40 years, with a slight female predominance. It is likely that the disease is the result of a genetic susceptibility predisposing to mounting an inappropriate immune response to viral infections. Viral infection has been postulated, however, none has been consistently detected or directly implicated in disease. Immunological mechanisms are central to disease pathogenesis and an active immunological response is present in areas of myelin loss. The cause of the immune response remains uncertain. An association with certain HLA antigens has been demonstrated.

2 Name and appearance of the lesions

The lesions of multiple sclerosis are confined to the brain and spinal cord. Areas of demyelination are termed 'plaques'.

- Areas of active recent demyelination appear as salmon-pink granular areas of softening in white matter. Histologically there is myelin loss associated with lymphocytic cuffing of small vessels. Macrophages enter the lesion and phagocytose the damaged myelin, accumulating lipid and forming foam cells. Astrocytes around plaque margins become enlarged.
- Areas of old myelin loss appear as sharply demarcated areas of firm, gelatinous, grey-pink discolouration. These inactive plaques, sometimes called burnt-out plaques, show loss of myelin, very few inflammatory cells and are occupied by astrocytes.

3 Blurred vision and eye pain

This is termed optic neuritis and is a very common manifestation of multiple sclerosis.

CASE 71

Mr Roderick Robertson, a 62-year-old coal miner, is seen because he has developed weakness of his left hand. On enquiry, he has been getting severe headaches over the past five weeks, often present when he wakes in the morning and made worse when he bends over. On examination, he has moderate weakness of his left arm and hand but no sensory changes. He has bilateral papilloedema. A CT scan shows a lesion about 3 cm in diameter in the right parietal lobe of the brain which enhances after contrast.

He is treated with dexamethasone and admitted to hospital a week later when he says that his headache has improved dramatically. A stereotactic biopsy of the lesion is perfomed and biopsy samples are sent for histology.

The pathology report reveals that the lesion is a glioblastoma multiforme. The tumour is composed of very pleomorphic astroglial cells with numerous mitoses. There is proliferation of vascular endothelium and extensive tumour necrosis.

Questions

1 How will this tumour behave clinically?
2 What is the prognosis?
3 Why was dexamethasone given prior to operation, leading to improvement in headache?

YOUR ANSWERS

1 Behaviour of tumour

2 Prognosis

3 Effects of dexamethasone

CASE 71 ANSWERS

p. 425

1 Behaviour of tumour

Glioblastomas are highly malignant astrocytic glial tumours with a rapid pace of growth. Like most gliomas, they diffusely infiltrate brain, and there is extensive local spread. With growth, tumour comes to occupy a significant volume of the brain and death is usually due to the effects of raised intracranial pressure.

2 Prognosis

There is a very poor prognosis with this type of tumour. There is a median survival of around 10 months from diagnosis.

3 Effects of dexamethasone?

Much of the swelling associated with brain tumours is the result of abnormally leaky blood vessels, causing cerebral oedema. Dexamethasone prevents this and reduces cerebral swelling, hence reducing intracranial pressure. In this case, the headache was due to raised intracranial pressure and improved when the peritumoural oedema was treated by dexamethasone.

CASE 72

Mr Tony Hope, a 39-year-old gas fitter, is admited to hospital because of rapidly progressive weakness. He developed an odd tingling in his feet and legs earlier in the day and this worsened, as did the weakness. He has now started to develop weakness in his arms. On examination, no reflexes can be elicited in the upper or lower limbs and there is generalized, moderate, flaccid muscle weakness. Sensory examination is normal, despite the tingling in his legs. Over the next five days, serial measurements of his respiratory function show that the weakness is affecting respiration. He is put on a ventilator.

Investigation	Result
Full blood count	Normal
Vitamin B$_{12}$	Normal
Neurophysiology	Markedly reduced conduction velocity in all nerves examined
CSF	Normal pressure, clear fluid. Mild increase in lymphoid cells and marked increase in protein. Sugar normal

Questions

1 What is the diagnosis?
2 What is the pathogenesis of this condition?
3 What is the prognosis?

YOUR ANSWERS

1 Diagnosis

2 Pathogenesis

3 Prognosis

CASE 72 ANSWERS

p. 430

1 Diagnosis

Guillain–Barré syndrome, or acute inflammatory polyradiculo-neuropathy. This is the commonest form of acute neuropathy. The marked slowing of conduction velocity in nerves is indicative of demyelination. The raised CSF protein supports the diagnosis.

2 Pathogenesis

This is is an immune-mediated demyelination of peripheral nerves, usually seen 2–4 weeks after a viral illness, but also triggered after a variety of infective processes. Histologically, nerves show infiltration by lymphoid cells with phagocytosis of myelin by macrophages. Patients have proximal as well as distal weakness because nerve roots are inflamed as well as peripheral nerves.

3 Prognosis

Widespread demyelination in peripheral nerves causes motor weakness, often leading to respiratory failure, with less prominent sensory changes. If patients are ventilated and carefully nursed, remyelination usually occurs over a period of several months, and is associated with recovery in most cases. Treatment with intravenous immunoglobulin in the acute phase of disease reduces the severity of disease and shortens the duration illness. Old age, the necessity for ventilatory support, and evidence of axonal degeneration on nerve conduction studies, are all adverse prognostic factors.

CASE 73

Commander Conrad Frimley–Blower RN is a retired naval commander, now aged 73. He has increasing weakness in his shoulders such that he finds it hard to lift his arms above his head. He has also developed weakness of his thighs and cannot pull himself up to stand unaided. On examination, he has moderate weakness in the shoulder and pelvic girdle muscles. He also has a slight ptosis. Investigations show a normal full blood count and ESR. His serum creatine kinase shows a very slight elevation above normal. Administration of a short-acting anticholinesterase drug has no benefit on his muscle strength.

A needle muscle biopsy is performed from the vastus lateralis and sent to the laboratory for enzyme histochemistry and histology. The pathology report reads as follows:

Needle biopsy of muscle: There is abnormal fibre size variation with many scattered atrophic fibres. A small number of fibres are necrotic and undergoing phagocytosis. There is a focal infiltrate of lymphoid cells. Several muscle fibres show rimmed vacuoles and eosinophilic inclusions. Electron microscopy shows that these inclusions are filamentous. The appearances are those of inclusion-body myositis.

Questions

1 What is the natural history of this disease?
2 What other inflammatory myopathies are there?
3 What are the reasons for administering anticholinesterase ?

CASE 73 ANSWERS p. 435

1 Natural history of inclusion-body myositis

Inclusion-body myositis is clinically similar to polymyositis but occurs mainly in elderly patients. Muscle biopsy shows inflammation of muscle, fibre necrosis and the presence of vacuoles and filamentous inclusions in fibres seen by electron microscopy. This disorder is important to diagnose as it is slowly progressive and, unlike other types of inflammatory myopathy, has a poor response to immunosuppressive treatment. This is an underdiagnosed condition.

2 Other types of inflammatory myopathy

Polymyositis presents clinically with weakness of proximal limb muscles, facial muscles, ptosis and dysphagia. Polymyositis may be associated with the presence of connective tissue diseases such as SLE, rheumatoid disease or scleroderma. and may also be a non-metastatic manifestation of malignancy. Dermatomyositis is clinically similar to polymyositis and includes the presence of a vasculitic skin rash. Sarcoid myopathy is an uncommon form of inflammatory muscle disease seen in sarcoidosis.

3 Reason for anticholinesterase

This clinical presentation could have been due to myasthenia gravis, a treatable condition caused by auto-antibodies directed to the acetylcholine receptors in motor end plates. Muscle strength transiently improves if anticholinesterase is administered. The usual drug given is edrophonium hydrochloride (Tensilon). Pretreatment with atropine (subcutaneous or intramuscular) is given to prevent the side effects of nausea and bradycardia.

13

OPHTHALMIC PATHOLOGY

CASE 74

Mr Bevis 'Sparky' Brown, a 58-year-old electrician, has been referred by his optician to the eye clinic. He has noticed some deterioration in his vision and, on checking by his optician, was found to have cupping of his optic disc. The pressure in his globe is measured by tonometry and found to be elevated, and a diagnosis of glaucoma is made. Examination of the iridocorneal angle shows that it is open with a normal anterior chamber.

Questions

1 What is the pathogenesis of primary open angle glaucoma?
2 What other types of glaucoma are there?
3 What is the natural history of untreated glaucoma?

YOUR ANSWERS

1 Pathogenesis of primary open-angle glaucoma

2 Other types of glaucoma

3 Natural history of untreated glaucoma

CASE 74 ANSWERS

p. 444

1 Pathogenesis of primary open angle glaucoma

Closing up of the trabecular meshwork (which normally leads to the canal of Schlemm), can occur as a degenerative process. It increases in incidence with age, being mainly encountered after the age of 40 and often being familial. Because the drainage angle is open, this is termed 'primary open-angle glaucoma'.

2 Other types of glaucoma

Glaucoma can be divided into primary and secondary groups:

- Primary open-angle glaucoma (see above).
- Primary closed-angle glaucoma develops in patients who have a congenitally shallow anterior chamber and who develop narrowing of the angle between the iris and the cornea, causing functional blockage to aqueous drainage. This particularly occurs when the pupil is dilated, as the iris thickens with contraction, hence acute attacks may be precipitated by being in the dark.
- Secondary closed angle glaucoma is caused by adhesions between the iris and cornea, for example, caused by uveitis or secondary to vascular proliferation due to retinal ischaemia.
- Secondary open-angle glaucoma is caused by blockage of the trabecular meshwork by particulate material in the aqueous – particularly degenerate lens material, pigment from melanocytic lesions, or macrophages accumulating in response to haemorrhage or inflammation.
- Congenital glaucoma is very rare, (seen in childhood with enlargement of the globe), and is mainly due to developmental defects in the drainage of aqueous.

3 Natural history of untreated glaucoma

The effects of raised intraocular pressure are cupping of the optic disc (detected on fundoscopy), and degeneration of retinal ganglion cells. Clinically, there is progressive peripheral visual field loss, leading to blindness in untreated cases. In acute glaucoma, there is breakdown of the endothelium leading to oedema of the cornea and formation of painful corneal bullae. In chronic glaucoma the sclera may stretch to form bulges termed 'staphylomas'.

14

ORTHOPAEDICS AND RHEUMATOLOGICAL PATHOLOGY

CASE 75

Mr Percy Treadgold, a 75-year-old retired gardener, is admitted with a painful thigh following trivial injury resulting from stumbling and falling whilst pushing a wheelbarrow load of fertilizer to his vegetable patch. He has had similar mild pain in the same thigh for some months, and also complains of back-ache; these symptoms have interfered with his normal garden-ing activities. The pain in his thigh on this last occasion is considerably more severe than he has experienced previously, and he is unable to move his right leg. X-ray shows a transverse fracture of the right mid-shaft of the femur; radiological abnormalities of the bone are noted at the site of fracture, and in the neck of the femur, the bone being irregularly lytic and sclerotic with the appearances of Paget's disease. Because of the history of minimal trauma, the unusual site of fracture, and the radiological abnormalities, pathological fracture is diagnosed. Further radiological investigation shows abnormal areas in the pelvic bones and in one lumbar vertebra.

The fracture is pinned and plated, and samples of abnormal bone from fracture site are taken, as well as a trephine biopsy from one of the abnormal areas in the iliac crest. The following laboratory investigations are undertaken:

Investigation	Result
Serum alkaline phosphatase	Markedly raised
Full blood count	No evidence of anaemia or white-cell abnormalities

Questions

1 What is the pathogenesis of Paget's disease?
2 What does the raised alkaline phosphatase indicate in this context?
3 What are the main effects of Paget's disease?
4 What abnormalities would the trephine biopsy of bone from the iliac crest have shown?

YOUR ANSWERS

1 Pathogenesis of Paget's disease

2 Significance of serum alkaline phosphatase

3 Effects of Paget's disease

4 Characteristic histological features of Paget's disease

CASE 75 ANSWERS

pp. 479, 480

1 Pathogenesis of Paget's disease

Paget's disease is of unknown cause. A viral infection of osteoclasts has been postulated, based on the finding of inclusions resembling paramyxovirus in cells.

2 Significance of serum alkaline phosphatase

In this context, the raised alkaline phosphatase is an indicator of increased bone formation due to increased osteoblast activity (osteoblasts are rich in alkaline phosphatase). An hepatic cause for raised alkaline phosphatase can be excluded by normal liver function tests. However, assays for bone-specific alkaline phosphatase are now available.

A markedly raised alkaline phosphatase is an indication for specific therapy with biphosphates or calcitonin. Other indicators are severe bone pain, hypercalcaemia and progressive deformity (with or without neurological defects).

3 Effects of Paget's disease

The main effects of Paget's disease are bone pain, bone deformity, hypercalcaemia and pathological fracture. Paget's disease also predisposes to the development of osteogenic sarcoma.

4 Characteristic histological features of Paget's disease?

- Increased osteoclastic resorption of bone by giant multinucleate osteoclasts.
- Increased new osteoid deposition by active cuboidal osteoblasts.
- New-bone formation shows woven pattern.
- There is marrow replacement with fibrous tissue.

CASE 76

Mrs Ravindra Patel, a 45-year-old lady, is brought to the hospital by her husband and mother because of increasing lack of mobility due to widespread bone pain and proximal muscle weakness. She is an immigrant from the Indian subcontinent, and is responsible for running the household and feeding her large family. She wears Indian national dress for her hospital attendance.

Investigation	Result
Serum calcium	Moderately reduced
Serum phosphate	Slightly reduced
Serum alkaline phosphatase	Raised
Bone X-ray	Generalized bone rarefaction with transverse linear bands in the cortical bone of the femora (Looser's zones)

Questions

1 What is the diagnosis?
2 What are the likely aetiological factors in this patient?
3 What do Looser's zones represent?
4 What other clinical chemistry investigations would be useful?

YOUR ANSWERS

1 Diagnosis

2 Aetiological in this case

3 Nature of Looser's zones

4 Other investigations

CASE 76 ANSWERS

pp. 478, 479

1 Diagnosis

This patient suffers from osteomalacia, due to defective mineralization of bone osteoid, usually the result of abnormalities in vitamin D. The symptoms of diffuse bone pain and proximal muscle weakness are characteristic, but osteomalacia is also a cause of pathological fracture.

2 Aetiology in this case

The two sources of vitamin D are dietary intake and vitamin D synthesis in the skin. In this woman, inadequate diet associated with inadequate synthesis of vitamin D in the skin are likely causes. Vitamin D synthesis requires exposure of the skin to ultraviolet light, and many women of her cultural background spend most of their time indoors and their traditional dress leaves very little skin exposed to ultraviolet light. Another cause could be malabsorption due to intestinal disease.

3 Nature of Looser's zones

Looser's zones represent microfractures which are common in the soft poorly mineralised bone of osteomalacia. Microfractures occur in both trabecular bone and in cortical bone, but only the latter are usually visible radiologically.

4 Other investigations

Although plasma 25-hydroxycholecalciferol estimations are possible, and are low in osteomalacia, they are not usually essential. However, it is always useful to exclude underlying chronic renal disease by performing simple renal function tests; remember that osteomalacia may follow chronic renal tubular failure because of the inability to convert vitamin D precursor to the active metabolite.

CASE 77

Ms Thea Dandridge, a slim, athletic, 32-year-old director of an avant-garde dance group, had become aware of discomfort (mainly stiffness) in the joints of her hands, particularly the knuckles, over the previous four weeks. The sensations are associated with soft-tissue swelling around the uncomfortable and sometimes painful joints. She has noticed that the symptoms are worst when she wakes up in the morning and improve during the day such that they do not interfere greatly with her profession. However, she has sought medical attention because she is beginning to experience similar discomfort from soft-tissue swelling and some reddening of the skin around her knees, greatly limiting her ability to perform. In addition, she has felt generally unwell, with lethargy and loss of appetite. On examination, there is swelling of the soft tissues around both knees, slight hyperaemia of the skin, with some limitation of movement by pain. There are similar, but less severe changes in the knuckles and proximal interphalangeal joints of the fingers, again associated with stiffness and limitation of movement. There are no other external abnormalities on examination, and the following investigations are performed :

Investigation	Result
Full blood count	Normocytic, normochromic anaemia
ESR	Moderately raised
Rheumatoid factor	Positive (high titre)
X-ray of fingers	Mild osteoporosis around the affected finger joints, associated with soft-tissue swelling

A diagnosis of rheumatoid disease is made and treatment is commenced. Her symptoms improve greatly and she is able to resume her profession for a time. However, her symptoms return intermittently, and she develops tender subcutaneous nodules around the elbow on the extensor surface.

Questions

1 What is the most significant and informative of the investigations above?
2 What is the explanation for the normocytic, normochromic anaemia?
3 What are the subcutaneous nodules around the elbow?

CASE 77 ANSWERS   pp. 490, 501, 502

1 Significant investigation

The presence of a positive rheumatoid factor in high titre indicates that this is rheumatoid arthritis rather than any of the other arthritides. It is positive in about 80% of cases. Rheumatoid factor is a circulating IgM autoantibody, and a high titre relates to clinical disease. Laboratory investigation may be performed by a Latex agglutination test, a Rose–Waaler test, as well as by specific radioimmunoassay and ELISA tests.

2 Reason for anaemia

A normocytic, normochromic anaemia is frequent, and is an example of the so-called 'anaemia of chronic illness'.

3 Nature of nodules

The nodules seen around the elbow are rheumatoid nodules: a frequent finding in active disease, particularly associated with high titre rheumatoid factor. They are composed of areas of degenerate collagen surrounded by a giant-cell granulomatous inflammatory response.

15

IMPORTANT MULTISYSTEM DISEASES

CASE 78

Mrs Amanda Strongbow is the 38-year-old publicity director for a charity that is dedicated to saving whales and dolphins. She is seen in the clinic for investigation. Over a six-month period, she has developed pains in her muscles and joints, felt generally unwell, and had crops of small ulcers in her mouth. She went to see her family doctor after a red skin rash developed on her face. The doctor noted proteinuria on a routine examination and has sent her for further investigations.

On examination, she has a red, slightly scaly rash on both cheeks and the bridge of her nose. A diagnosis of systemic lupus erythematosus is made

Investigation	Result
Full blood count	Lymphopenia
ESR	Moderately elevated
Serum urea and electrolytes	Normal
Serum albumin	Reduced
24-hour urine protein	Greatly elevated
Anti-double-stranded DNA	High titre

Questions

1 What is the reason for the proteinuria and how can it be investigated?
2 What haematological abnormalities may be seen in SLE?
3 Is the skin rash relevant?

1 Reason for proteinuria and investigation

2 Haematological abnormalities

3 Relevance of skin rash

CASE 78 ANSWERS p. 498

1 Reason for proteinuria and investigation

Renal involvement in lupus is common. Lupus nephritis may show many different patterns, mimicking other forms of glomerular abnormality.

- Focal segmental mesangial glomerulonephritis.
- Focal segmental proliferative glomerulonephritis with tuft damage.
- Membranous nephropathy pattern.
- Membranoproliferative pattern.

Glomerular damage is caused by the deposition of immune complexes in the glomerulus. The complexes may be deposited in the basement membrane (leading to basement-membrane thickening), or in the mesangium (leading to mesangial expansion); immunofluorescence methods show that the immune complexes contain three types of immunoglobulin, IgG, IgA and IgM, and two types of complement, C3 and C1Q. Renal biopsy is an important investigation in SLE with renal involvement.

2 Haematological abnormalities

- A normocytic hypochromic anaemia.
- An autoimmune haemolytic anaemia (approx 10%) with red-cell antibodies and positive Coomb's test.
- Reduced peripheral white-cell count, usually due to disproportionate reduction of lymphocytes (lymphopenia).
- Thrombocytopenia – -sometimes associated with the presence of antiplatelet antibodies.
- Predisposition to thrombosis – particularly if there are antiphospholipid/lupus anticoagulant antibodies.

3 Relevance of skin rash

The skin rash is one of the diagnostic features of SLE, although there are other skin manifestations of the disease.

CASE 79

Mrs Maisie Wyles is the 67-year-old wife of a car mechanic. She has come to see you because of deteriorating vision in her right eye. On examination, she is moderately overweight and ophthalmoscopic examination reveals a cataract in the right eye. The fundus of the left eye is visible, and shows hard exudates, haemorrhages and microaneurysms. Routine testing shows glycosuria and moderate proteinuria. A random blood sugar is elevated at 8 mmol/l. There is mild elevation of serum urea and creatinine levels. A urine sample that was sent for culture, later shows that she does not have a urinary tract infection. A diagnosis of diabetes mellitus is made.

Questions

1 What type of diabetes mellitus does she have?
2 What is the pathogenesis of this type of diabetes mellitus.
3 What do the changes in the fundus signify, and what other changes need to be looked for on follow-up?
4 What pathological changes will be present in the kidneys to cause the proteinuria?

YOUR ANSWERS

1 Type of diabetes

2 Pathogenesis of this type of diabetes

3 Changes in the fundus, and other changes to look for

4 Cause of the proteinuria

CASE 79 ANSWERS
pp. 505, 507

1 Type of diabetes

There are three main types of diabetes mellitus: **Type I diabetes** (insulin-dependent diabetes mellitus – IDDM, or juvenile onset diabetes); **Type II diabetes** (non-insulin-dependent diabetes – NIDDM, or maturity onset diabetes) and **secondary diabetes** which is secondary to disease of the pancreas or is caused by hormones which antagonize the effects of insulin, for example, in Cushing's syndrome and acromegaly. In this case the patient probably has Type II diabetes.

2 Pathogenesis of this type of DM

The precise pathogeneses in Type II diabetes are not known, although aetiological factors such as age, obesity and a genetic predisposition are well-recognized. There is a strong genetic factor since between 90–100% of identical twins show concordance. Inheritance is considered to be polygenic.

3 Changes in the fundus, and other changes to look for

The fundal changes are those of background retinopathy due to small vessel abnormalities in the retina (hard exudates, haemorrhages and microaneurysms). This does not usually affect acuity. Other changes that occur as a result of diabetes are:

- Proliferative retinopathy – in which there is extensive proliferation of new small blood vessels in the retina. Sudden deterioration in vision can result from vitreous haemorrhage from the proliferating new vessels or from the development of retinal detachment.
- Maculopathy is caused by oedema, hard exudates or retinal ischaemia in the cone-rich macula, causing marked reduction in acuity.
- Cataract formation is greatly increased in diabetics.
- Glaucoma shows an increased incidence in diabetics due to neovascularisation of the iris, rubeosis iridis.

4 Cause of proteinuria

The kidney are often abnormal in diabetes. Renal glomerular lesions cause proteinuria. There may be:

- Glomerular basement membrane thickening.
- Diabetic glomerulosclerosis, both diffuse and nodular.
- Glomerular exudative lesions.

There is eventual glomerular loss through hyalinization, causing chronic renal failure. In addition there is predisposition to urinary tract infection with risk of papillary necrosis, and tendency to chronic ischaemia associated with severe atherosclerosis and arteriolosclerosis.

CASE 80

Mr Cuthbert O'Grady is a 48-year-old man, who is registered disabled because of severe ankylosing spondylitis. Despite his disability and poor mobility, he still manages to do a lot of fund raising for local charities. He still gets a lot of pain from his disease, but this is reasonably controlled with non-steroidal anti-inflammatory drugs which he takes regularly. He has been feeling increasingly tired lately and comes to see you for a check-up.

Investigation	Result
Full blood count	Mild normochromic anaemia
ESR	Greatly elevated
Urea	Moderately elevated
Creatinine	Moderately elevated
Sodium	Normal
Potassium	Normal
Urinalysis	Heavy proteinuria

He is referred to a renal physician to investigate the cause of his proteinuria. His kidneys are slightly reduced in size and, after further tests, a renal biopsy is performed. This reveals thickening of glomerular basement membrane and walls of renal arterioles by amyloid.

Questions

1 What type of amyloid is likely to be present?
2 What are the main sites for secondary amyloid deposition?
3 How else may amyloid be diagnosed?
4 What is the commonest type of amyloid?

YOUR ANSWERS

1 Type of amyloid

2 Main sites for amyloid deposition

3 Diagnosis

4 Commonest type of amyloid

CASE 80 ANSWERS   pp. 509, 510

1 Type of amyloid

The amyloid is most likely to be derived from serum amyloid-A protein, an acute-phase protein produced by the liver in response to his inflammatory spondyloarthopathy.

2 Main sites for amyloid deposition

The main sites for amyloid deposition are kidney, heart, nerves, liver, spleen, and gut.

3 Diagnosis

The diagnosis of systemic amyloidosis is usually confirmed by tissue biopsy. The most useful site for biopsy is the rectal mucosa where amyloid can be detected in the submucosal vessels in 60–70% of cases of generalized amyloidosis. Amyloid may also be detected in renal biopsies or liver biopsies.

More recently, radiolabelled serum amyloid-P can be injected into patients and imaged, when it localizes to any amyloid deposits.

4 Commonest type of amyloid

The commonest example of amyloid deposition is in the brain in normal ageing and also in Alzheimer's disease. The amyloid is derived from a normal neuronal membrane protein termed Alzheimer Precursor Protein (APP), being formed from a peptide fragment termed β-protein or A4 protein.

INDEX